911 Emergency Safety Manual for women

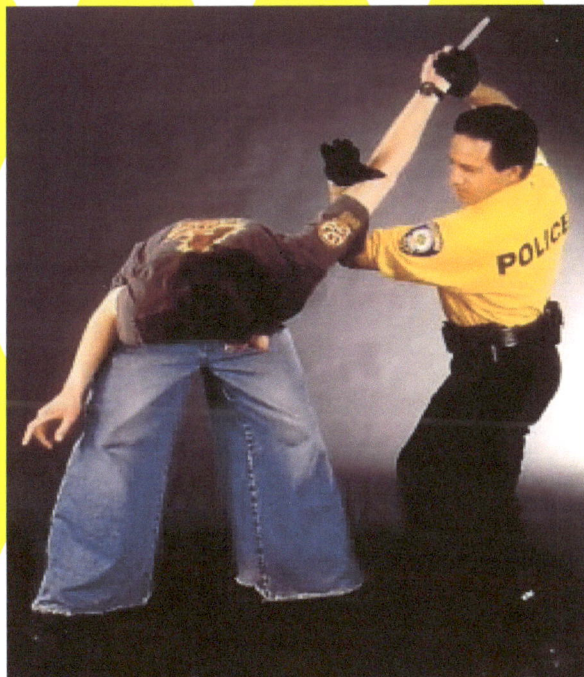

This reference may save your Life and The Secrets will make you 98% Safer

NOW !

Table of Contents

911 Emergency Safety Manual

C.Heimlich Ph.D.

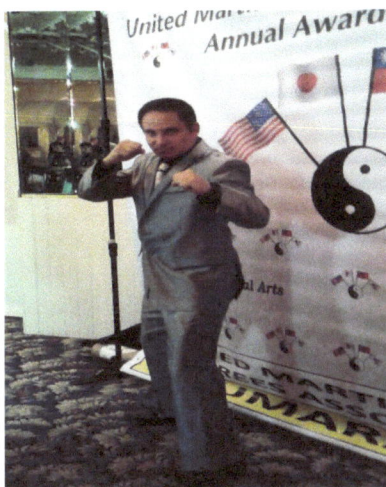

The most important book you will ever have or need! The information and self Defense Tactical Maneuvers that are listed have been broken down for easy learning and application. Start out very slow to learn the moves then put them together and apply them with some effort, not to harm your partner, but to make sure they work. Practice over and over until they are like 2nd nature!

OK, now lets get busy !

I would like to thank all of you who believed in me and helped me to become what I am today. My many students, past ,present and future from whom I've learned so much, and that I will continue to learn from ,as there is so much more to learn!

Education is Power !

And to all my friends and Family who gave me strength to continue the Journey.

Thank you all ,

Yours in Safety,
C.Heimlich Ph.D.
A.K.A. Dr. Protection

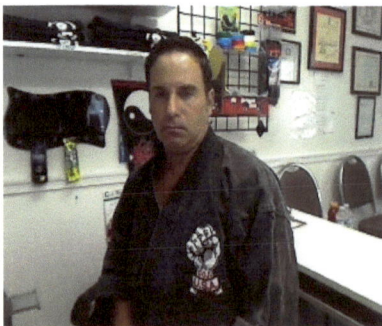

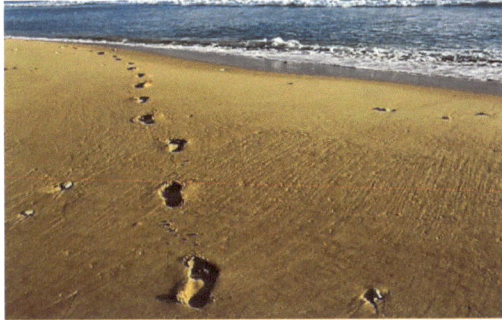

"A journey of a thousand miles begins with a first step".

Welcome to your first step. As with all first steps you must learn to start out slow and take your time! Read and put this life saving material into effect immediately! Be careful not to ever be over confident!

Your journey should be serious, but enjoyable and educational.

I would say good luck, but there is no such thing as LUCK only OPPORTUNITY!

So lets get started!

Understand this manual is designed to help save you or your family from serious harm, or even death. Please note, it is not intended to frighten, it is intended to Educate. I must however warn you that this book contains serious adult subject matter with graphic information, and details. Please keep an open mind in order to understand and absorb this Vital Life Saving information!

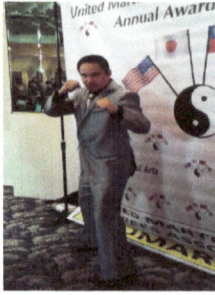

About the Author

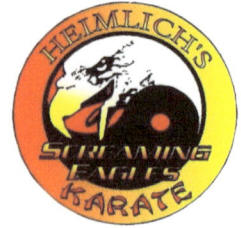

C. Heimlich Ph.D.

Dr. C. Heimlich, Ph.D., also known as Dr. Protection, started professional training in 1982, and quickly became a Champion Competitor. He has been recognized for his passion and ability and has received many awards since opening his first School in Southern N.J..

He received a master level Certification, along with a Bachelors Degree from Dr. Peter Urban, the Grand Patriarch of all Goju Ryu Karate in America.

He is a multiple Martial Arts Hall of fame inductee. In 2010, he was presented the Silver 25 year lifetime achievement award. The award was presented by, actor/Martial arts professional Michael Jai White, and the famous Don the Dragon Wilson. Over the years he has had many other inductions presented to him by many other celebrity Martial Artists. In 2018 he was honored by action Magazine Hall of Honors.

Dr. Heimlich is a Shichidan 7th Degree Black belt. He is also a former police officer, an author, a motivator, an actor ,a speaker, an innovator, and an inspirational leader. Dr. Protection is a certified fitness instructor, and personal trainer. He received a PhD in Martial Sciences and Philosophy. However, today he is the founder and Director of the Dr. Protection Personal Protection Safety Center. He conducts seminars, workshops and demonstrations. He has trained with some of the Greatest and most Famous Martial artist in the world ,such as, his Sensei, **The Late Dr. Peter Urban**, **The Late Undefeated World Heavy Weight Champion Joe Lewis** , **The Founder of Sin Moo Hapkido, Ji Han Jae,** as well as many others. He continues to teach and educate Women on Personal Protection and other related Issues. He is available for seminars, workshops, speaking engagements , acting and stunt work and other small bits .

This could be the most important book you could ever own! It is a must for every Woman!

There are 62 pages of some of the most life saving, life enhancing information ever compiled!

What he has done, is give the reader some of his valuable and useable knowledge based on information from his many years of study, training and teaching. He is positive this book will be one of the most important books you can have in your possession! He takes this very seriously and hopes you will too!

Dr. Protection has spent his entire life time working on these and many other issues, not only for Women, but for Children and Men. The bottom line is , that every one should learn Martial Arts! I'm not saying you should be the next Kata champion or Weapons expert, but that all should have a Basic Foundation of Personal Protection.

Eventually a level of understanding will be achieved and techniques will be performed perfectly, time after time. This takes time so be very patient , never give up. I have purposely kept most of the techniques in this book as simple to do as possible. There are many more and they become much more complicated and difficult to learn. At that point you will need a partner to practice with ,do not be afraid ,you will not hurt them .Practice slow at first ,then learn to apply the technique as illustrated .You will not injure anyone ,including your self ,due to the escape and compliance nature of these movements .So keep this in mind do not allow your partner to just let go of you, or even hold you in a less than real hold . All of these techniques work . They must be as real as possible , if you struggle at first don't give up you will learn to overcome your suspicions and gain the I can't do it attitude. Again I urge you to never give in or have poor attitude! You can and will be very successful with all this information provided. Concentrate and Focus, believe in your self and remember, train with the mind set this is the real thing! It needs to be real so that, God forbid ,you are ever in a real life or death situation it will feel the same ,this is how you learn to conquer fear and over come your adversary .

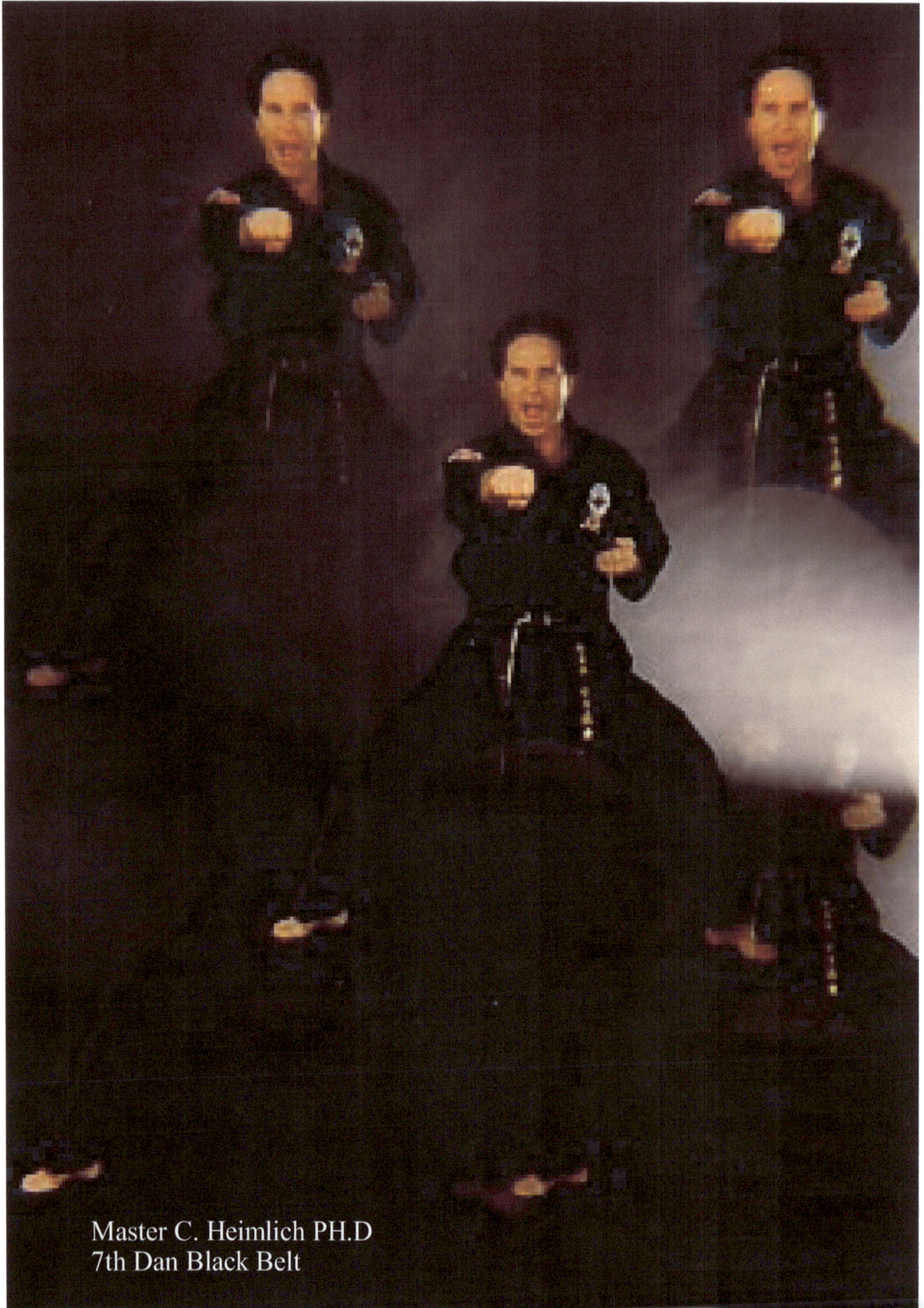

Master C. Heimlich PH.D
7th Dan Black Belt

Master Heimlich,(Dr. Protection) would like to dedicate this book ,to all those who have suffered the loss of a loved one, or had to endure the brutal violence of a violent crime.

He knows and believes, that with the commitment to personal protection we can change the outcome of violent crimes!

ONE CRIME AT A TIME!

We now live in the most violent society on earth! The Center on disease control has now declared murder as an epidemic!

We must stop this violence! We must put an end to it. He believes we can make a difference , as like anything else , by educating the general public on these issues and making everyone aware of the seriousness!

Personal Protection , Karate and the Martial Arts in general have received bad reputations due to the many myths and fallacies portrayed on the T.V. and in the movies. The misconceptions and mysteries surrounding the Martial Arts, need to cleared up and corrected.

People still approach Master Heimlich,(Dr. Protection) and ask him if he had to register his hands with the police as a deadly weapon. He always asks them," did you register your mouth as a deadly weapon, because your words are killing me!"

Seriously, we need to change the perception of what Martial arts training is. Some people view it as a sport , or a fitness routine. Some say its to learn how to fight. Some say it's a baby sitting service, others say its dangerous and violent. Well guess what, they are all wrong! MA is a way of life that creates awareness, strengthens, self worth, self esteem, gives balance, control , emotional, spiritual, and physical components that nothing else can offer. . Not to mention discipline, and respect and, oh yeah……... …………………....*Self defense!*

KARATE

This is life enhancing, life saving , street smart, self protection , however this is of course, the last resort . We try to avoid confrontations as much as possible ,we try to walk away ,we try to avoid certain circumstances ,we try to keep our opinions to our selves and all for good cause.

This is the true essence of Martial Arts .Why, you ask ? Again, because it's a way of life, its about Discipline and respect .We know that we can cause damage and so for this reason we save it for only an extreme emergency. When no other choice is available that's when we strike with every thing we have , every thing we been taught and had practiced for , this and only this is the time to execute what you know.

I can tell you first hand, and not to brag ,but to educate you, I have used my training several times . I have been in many life or death situations and was able to execute my techniques with precision and accuracy and effortlessly to take out my opponent . Therefor I know what I'm talking about I have survived Knife and Gun attacks while being weaponless myself and survived it all without incident . Otherwise I would not be reading this book .

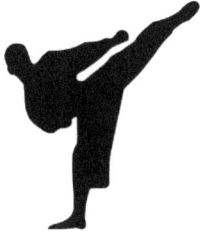

MAIN OBJECTIVE

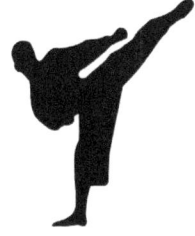

In this emergency Manual, you will learn the Secrets of Personal Protection, as offered by the Official leading Expert, Dr. Protection!

His objective is to give the reader the necessary tools for personal Protection in an easy to understand and easy to follow format without the unnecessary hype and false information that you may get from most personal protection courses, and books.

This is a real to life tool kit complete with all the basic tools. When put together it can and will save your life. He is very passionate about teaching and writing. He will not sacrifice or water down material in order to stretch it out or make it something it is not. He promises no false sense of security or false hope. What he does give you is a lesson plan for action. It is complete with tactical training, and practical street-smart personal, and family protection lessons. With all the insights to alertness, awareness, criminal psychology, and other life saving attributes, this manual provides the reader with critical life saving skills.

When finally memorized and practiced, it will indeed provide you with a new found sense of security and confidence that you can use immediately!

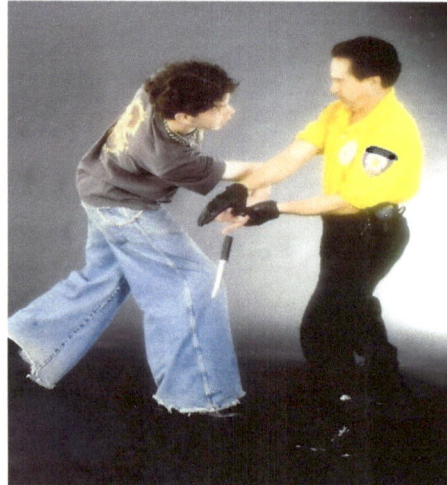

The Secret to Becoming

98 % SAFER

Is now in your hands! This secret alone is worth more than any monetary value.

You need to ask yourself a Question. If you were faced by a Vicious Criminal who had a gun to your head, and told you to prepare to die, how much money would you be willing to pay to have the knowledge and the know how to be back at home at that particular moment? To be safe and alive with your family and friends.

Many people have been in that exact predicament and found themselves begging for their life just moments before it was brutally taken away!

Did you know, you have a greater chance of being a victim of a violent crime than being in a car accident? Can you really do something about this? Yes indeed you can, and you have chosen this manual as a first step in that quest! Your safety is your right! When it comes down to personal protection, we really only have 2 choices. You can either throw up your hands give up and pray that nothing ever happens to you, or you can take charge of your life and educate yourself to prevent being a victim all together . I believe, as should you ,the latter is the more realistic decision . This Manual is not meant to scare you, but rather meant to educate you. So please Read and Study this material with an open mind. Understand the seriousness and don't be delusional or ever think nothing like that could ever happen to you. Don't live in Denial!

CRIME CLOCK:

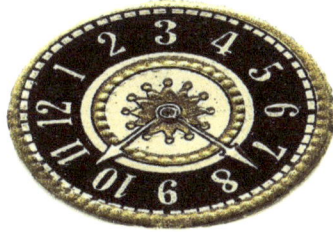

- A women is raped every 46 seconds in America….That's 78 rapes each hour!
- Every day, four women are killed by their abusive husbands.
- 25% of girls, and 17% of boys will be sexually assaulted by the time they are 18 years old.
- 14% of all American women acknowledge having been violently abused by a husband or boyfriend.
- From 1992 to 1993 29% of all violence against women by a lone offender was by an intimate.
- 75% of domestic homicides occur after the victim has left the perpetrator.
- 28% of all homicides of women are domestic violence related.
- 95% of reported domestic assaults, the female is the victim, and the male is the perpetrator.
- 75% of every rape is committed by a man that the victim knows.
- 25% of rapes take place in a public area or a parking garage.

These shocking facts show that violent crimes can affect anyone at any-time, regardless of where they live or work. Theses crimes include assault, domestic violence, robbery, car jacking, rape and murder.

Based on theses statistics, its possible that at some point in your life you might be a victim of a violent crime.

The criminal's primary strategy is to use the advantage of surprise. Criminals mainly choose targets which appear to be unaware of their sur-rounding. So please be prepared before something happens!

More crime clock statistics :

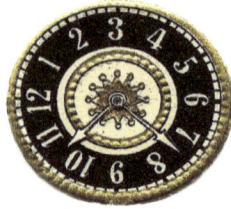

- 25% of rapes take place in a parking garage or public area.
- 63% of rapes occur between 6 pm and 6am.
- Victims received injuries in over 47% of all rapes.
- More than 50% of rapists were under the influence of drugs or alcohol when committing their crime.
- Over 80% of assaults were committed without the use of a weapon.

Age Rape/Sexual Assault statistics:

- 15% of rape victims are under the age of 12
- 29% of rape victims are between the ages of 12 and 17
- 44% of rape victims are under the age of 18
- 80% of rape victims are under the age of 30

Robbery Statistics:

- 71% of robberies were committed by strangers
- More than 50% of robberies happened between 6 pm and 6 am
- Over 65% of robberies used a weapon to complete their crime.

Awareness skills

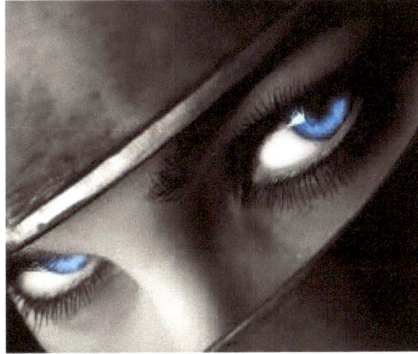

The Statistics that you had just read are conservative and yet, are getting worse! What can be done to slow them down and make them the exception, instead of the rule? Many of these violent acts could have been prevented if only the Victim were more Aware. In TNT Dr. Protection teaches that there are 3 Categories of **Awareness**.

Criminal Awareness , Situational Awareness and Self Awareness

Criminal awareness -involves the understanding of the Nature and Dynamics of the criminals as well as their Motives ,Methods, and Capabilities.
Study the local news and media for criminal activity, then answer
Who ,What, Where, When, Why, and How.
Theses exercises will begin to reveal valuable information.

There are 3 Rapist Profiles in criminal awareness

Power Rapist
- Full of doubt
- Wants victim to engage
- Often a stalker
- Well educated white collar
- Relatively easy to defend

Anger
- Angry and Hateful
- Blames Women for life's problems
- Uses profanity and abusive language
- Strikes spontaneously
- Physically assaults victim
- Highly Dangerous

Sadistic
- Enjoys Bizarre and devious acts
- Enjoys torture and intimidation
- Likely to kidnap victim
- May mutilate victim
- Extremely Dangerous

Special Relations

Date Rape and Date Rape Drugs, are a newer form of rape that are quickly becoming more and more common, as well as Dangerous!
When out on a date be **cautious**, and **remain alert**.
Do not drink to get drunk!
Have a friend that you trust to be close by. **Observe what you eat and what you drink!**
Do not leave your drink unattended
If your date seems to be getting **out of control, dominating, abusive or violent,**
Leave with some one else. **Be very cautious of your actions. Be discrete**
Not to escalate the situation or endanger yourself or some one else!

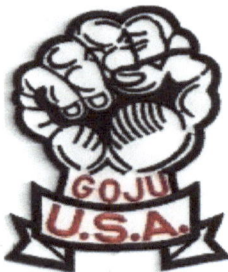 *Situational Awareness*

Is basically total alertness, presence and focus on your surroundings!
You must train your senses to detect and assess people, places, objects and actions that can pose a danger. Too many times we lack the ability to heighten awareness, this is due to the conserved belief that nothing can happen to me syndrome, and to our ever growing busy lifestyles.

Denial, and the every day pressures of life interfere with the perception of danger that lurk all around us! If you do not pay attention to these hidden dangers, your chances of becoming a victim, are greatly increased!

We have this misconception that criminals are stupid and incompetent, on the contrary they are shrewd, bold, and dominant. They are also excellent at observing human behavior, and capable of assessing body language, walk, talk, and state of mind. They know what to look for and how to exploit it.

They are also selective predators. They will for example, engage you in conversation to assess your weaknesses, and evaluate your apprehension, fear, and awareness. They are looking for an easy strike or what they call a "VIC". As you increase your awareness, you send out a different, new signal. One of confidence and strength. This is the message you want them to perceive!

Congratulations you are on your way to becoming 98 % SAFER!

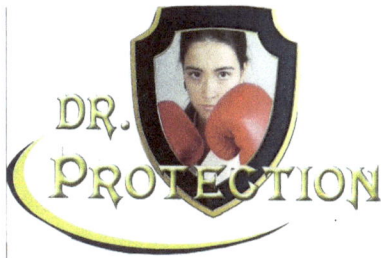

SELF AWARENESS

Self *awareness contains many physical attributes. Self awareness has many different attributes and skills. So first we need to know, do we really know ourselves? What aspects of yourself would provoke violence? Which of any would promote a proper reaction in self defense? Look at certain aspects important to self protection and ask yourselves a few questions.*

Physical attributes - *What are your physical strengths? What are your weaknesses? Are you overweight or underweight? Does your body language tell a story of who you are? Do you think you provoke or deter a violent attack? Do you have any training in self defense? Are you fit or out of shape? Do you have the skill to disarm a wheeling attacker? Do you smoke or drink?*

 Mental attributes- *What are your mental strengths and weaknesses? Are you an optimist or a pessimist? Do you have confidence or are you fearful? Are you insecure? How do you handle stress? Do you Panic or frighten easily? Do you have any phobias? (Communication skills), What are your strengths and weaknesses in expressing yourself with words? Are you easy to aggravate? Can you diffuse a hostel situation? Are your words and your voice in the pitch and tone and volume all under control? Can you communicate adequately under stress.*

 Personality Traits- *What type of person are you? Are you passive or aggressive? Are you opinionated, argumentative? Are you open minded? Are you fiery or loud ? Are you quiet or calm? Are you quick to anger? Do you hold grudges? Are you sensitive to remarks or statements? Do you lose your temper easily?*

Gender and age- *Note the different types of violent crimes that are directed towards you because of your gender or your age. Understand who's more likely to become of a victim of a certain crime. Understand your weaknesses and your vulnerabilities due to your age.*

Occupation - *Does your occupation make you vulnerable to different forms of violence? Are you involved in the law enforcement? Are you a celebrity? Are you in politics? Do you carry large sums of money? Are you a likely target for kidnapping or terrorism?*

Income level- *Note what types of crimes are directed towards you because of your income. Are you wealthy? Are you poor? Does your financial situation force you to live in poor neighborhoods? Are you flashy? Do you show evidence of wealth? How do you live ? These are just a few of the many Questions you need to ask your self in evaluating your Self Awareness.*

17

Conquering Fear

We are born with two fears , one is the fear of falling ,

the other is the fear of loud noises!

The other fears that we develop, come from different experiences that we have as small children and or when faced with tragic incidents.

So for the purpose of this book we will only discuss the fear of being a victim.

Fear is a crippling emotion that will leave you totally defenseless, unless you learn a few secrets.

We must understand how this type of fear effects the human body physiologically. The heart begins to beat faster and faster, the nose flares to allow more oxygen to the lungs, the brain also compensates for the horrific events unfolding. The muscles begin to get weaker and the brain starts to shut down. This is natures way of preparing for the violent act .

My analogy to over come this fear is ;

"Fear is like fire"

Is fire good or bad?

Fear is like fire! When out of control it destroys, burns down buildings and kills! However, when fire is controlled, its good and useful . It cooks our food, heats our homes, and gives us light. So once controlled, fear like fire, can be utilized to help you survive a situation. So it is ok to be afraid, but you must control it. Once this is understood and this emotion is under control, you can take personal protection to the next level. In order to control fear you must train and practice all the components of personal protection until self confidence is in place verses anxiety, confusion, and uncertainty. This will allow you to make important life saving choices without delay and with proper timing .

When the window of opportunity presents itself you must be ready and able to act upon it .

Emotion

Did you know there are over 900 emotions associated with the human psyche? Socrates, once said "know thyself". These are the most profound two words in all of humanity. For we all believe we know ourselves, but do we really? The average person can name just a handful or more of these emotions. So how can we truly understand who we are? To slay the dragon, we must know the dragon!

The criminal works in a similar way. To prevent being a victim we must understand the criminal. The criminal uses what we call street smarts. They know how to use reverse psychology. They know how to play on your emotions. They look for weaknesses as well as strengths. They look for awareness, as well as alertness. They are also opportunistic and will take advantage of the first window of opportunity that presents itself. When accessing a situation, all these things must be taken in to account. This in part is the beginning of personal protection.

Also, when looking for a victim, the assailant will use strategies to create the scenario they are looking for. They will use verbal cues, as well as body language in communicating what they want or expect. When approached by a stranger, it is ok and wise to tell that person **STOP!!!** You may then tell that person to keep their distance. If that person gets upset or angry over your request, then you know that that person has bad intentions, and they will begin to use guilt. Never let down your guard, and never feel guilty about speaking your mind, due to the fact that this is your personal space and your private space. No one has a right to violate that space. When you begin to exercise your rights, you begin to be less vulnerable!!
You show strength and confidence, this in turn will send out a different message about who you are. Be sure to always walk with pride and self confidence. Be aware of you body language ,send out positive signals!
Always be in control but, be careful not to be over confident or to let down your guard at any time!

Personal Protection

In order to be able to Protect yourself, or a loved one successfully, You must first learn all the attributes that had led you to this point. Then, and only then, will you be able to except, understand and take control of your Person in order to meet and exceed this new Secret.

The Physical Self

Yes, you will need to be in some form of physical fitness in order to be able to defend yourself.   This will greatly enhance your probabilities of stopping or surviving an all out attack.

Now, lets take into account a few things;

First, the average man has the strength of a 12 year old boy.

Second, The average man has about a 2 minute endurance limit. These are very important things to know. Do not underestimate your adversary. Some criminals actually train to be stronger so that they will be more successful.

Self Defense
Exercises

If you already exercise or belong to a gym, you may continue to do your own work out. However, if you do not already have an exercise plan or routine you may start here. You may even want to seek out a professional fitness trainer.

This is part of my own personal routine. Hope you like it!

For the beginner ;
First of all, do not except walking as a form of exercise. It is a form of locomotion only! You will benefit from these exercises. You should start out slow, or you may add / subtract to whatever level you want to begin. However, I recommend to start in this order ;

Push-ups: Begin with **10** and work your way up to **60 –80** according to your ability.

*Sit -ups:*___As many as possible until you can reach **100**

Leg Extensions : Lay on your back. Pick knee up with legs folded until knee is parallel to the floor. Then extend legs from the knee down to the foot. Next bring knee to shoulder and extend entire leg straight out to side same amount, **10** each. Then kick back with the heal, extend back and hold leg as high as possible for **10** seconds.
Sit-ups– As many as possible until **100.** Jumping and kicks, work your way up to **100.** Stretching—**10** minutes

Next :Turn over on back with legs pulled in close to chest. Extend legs out fully and keep feet off the floor 6 inches. Hold for 2 seconds, then fold legs back in slow motion. Complete as many as possible until you reach 15.
Next: do the same as above but when extended open legs wide. Then close together and retract back, same form.
Next: start with legs fully extended, open and close same amount.

Do not cheat, strain or hold breath!
For proper form check out our website: heimlichskarate.com

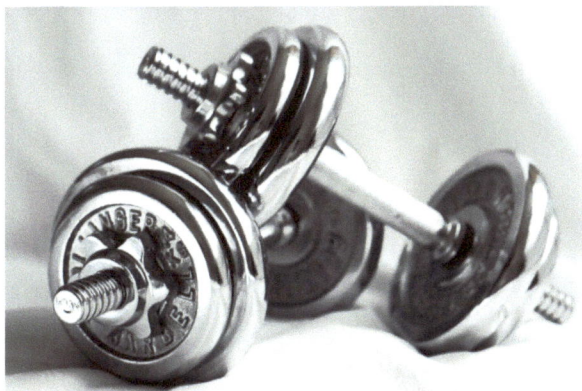

Don't feel like going to the gym? With these fat burning exercises, you don't even need a gym membership ,or even any equipment for that matter.

The best workouts are always going to be those that consist of moves that engage multiple large muscle groups. You can easily take a simple, conventional toning move and turn it into a something more efficient that gives you the most bang for your buck for every moment that you spend on your workout.

For example, consider the **bicep curl**. It is an extremely effective basic strength training or toning movement, however, 3 sets of them is not exactly going to crank up your calorie burning furnace or cancel out that cheeseburger and microbrew you had for dinner last night. Instead of isolating just the bicep, you could combine the move with a lunge to significantly boost the caloric burn, and simultaneously tone your lower body.

Apply the above concept to the exercises that make up your routines and they become dynamic, fat burning workouts.
Here are the best examples that put this principle to work.;

Top 10 Best Fat Burning Exercises

1 **Burpees** - This at home cardio move tones your core, upper body and legs all at once- it's a triple threat exercise that everyone tends to dread for good reason; they are hard! But they also work.

2 **Jumping Lunges** - Lunges are a fantastic thigh toning exercise; add in the momentum required to jump up in between lunges and the move turns into an incredible calorie burner.

3 **Pilates Leg Pulls** - Tone your core, gluteus, and thighs with this one simple Pilates move. Because all of the large muscle groups involved, you burn a high number of calories while you are toning.

4 **Jackknife Crunches** - Jackknife Crunches are an advanced abdominal move that engage both the upper and lower abs for maximal toning in the least amount of time. They are especially beneficial because lower abs can be hard to target without equipment.

5 **Lunges with Reverse Leg Raise** - This tones the gluts., thighs, oblique's, and lower back, all while building coordination and balance.

6 **Jumping Squats** - Do this exercise for a minute or two straight and you wont have any doubts about how challenging it is. This plyometric is also great for building explosive speed.

7 **Push Ups** - Push ups are a total body exercise that are easily modified and can be made to be very challenging, even for the most avid exerciser. If a regular push up feels too easy for you, try the Single Leg Push Up.

8 **Side Planks with Leg Raises** - While this most specifically targets the outer thighs, oblique's, and deltoids, it requires the strength and coordination of the entire body to hold up the base Pilates side plank.

9 **Mountain Climbers** - Mountain Climbers can feel like a punishment, but they truly are one of the best overall toning and fat burning moves out there that don't require a bit of equipment.

10 **Jumping Jacks** - This simple at home cardio essential is an excellent way to get your heart rate up quickly. Add it in between strength training sets to keep your caloric burn high.

Tactical Choices

The next secret is understanding and acknowledging what your tactical choices are.

In any given situation, you have 5 Tactical choices , <u>ONLY</u> !

Choice # 1 *De-escalate* - Taking an out of control situation and, bringing it under control using the pitch , tone, and volume of your voice as a deterrent. To do this you must remain calm and soft spoken.   The quieter you are, the quieter they will become. For they can't hear you over their loud obnoxious voice.

Choice #*2* *Assertive* - Stand your ground! Be strong! Do not use profanity! But be stern, strong, and loud. Keep command! Say No! Say it with Authority and Mean it , never show Fear !

Choice #3 *Comply* - Do what they ask, and give them what they want. However, there is a trick to this. If they command you to give them something, and no other choice is applicable, than do so. However, throw it opposite of your escape route.

Choice #4 *Escape* - Walk away, run away , get out of there!

Choice #5 Self Defense - Last and final choice, FIGHT back!

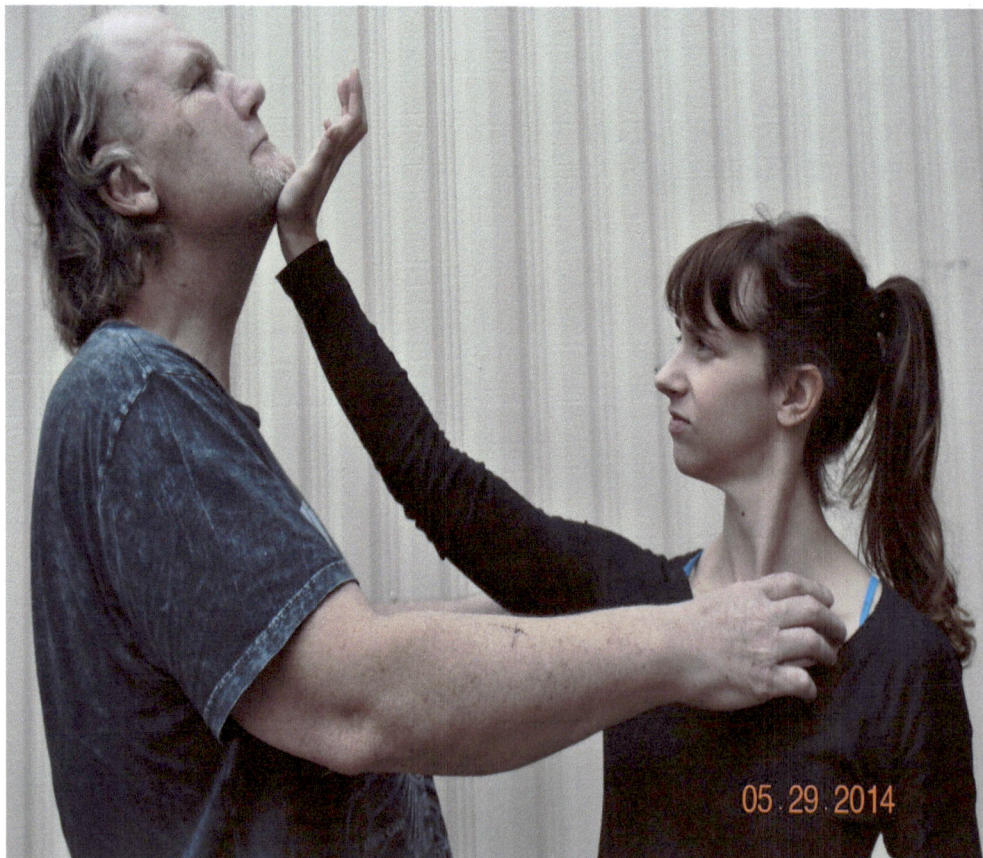

05.29.2014

On the next few pages, you will learn some Basic Self defense Techniques that I have kept as simple to learn as possible . I tried to take out the complication so that these can be practiced, and learned easily.

But you must try and learn them , then put them to use with different people until you feel confident and comfortable with them . You must know them inside and out!

Remember the old saying , "Practice makes Perfect ",well that's actually incorrect ! Only "PERFECT PRACTICE" makes perfect ! So practice these every day, it doesn't take long. I'm not asking you to dedicate your day to them, just 15 to 20 min a day. You may spend more time with them if you like, and when you realize what you can do, you will want to do them more often. You may even show your friends, but be carful , you never know who your enemy is, or will become. They say keep your friends close and your enemies closer. Only trouble with this is , that sometimes you can't tell the difference!

This is a side kick against a side grab ,the opponent grabs you from an angle or side ,then you chamber the leg to perform a side kick ,the opponent will not expect this as they lose control and fall as a result .

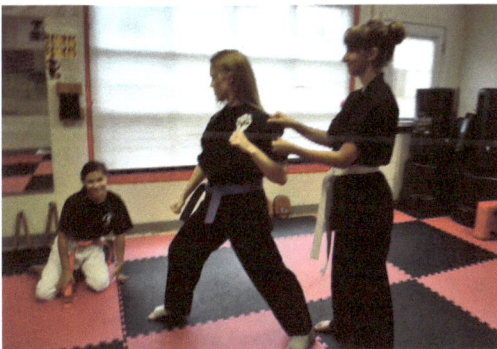

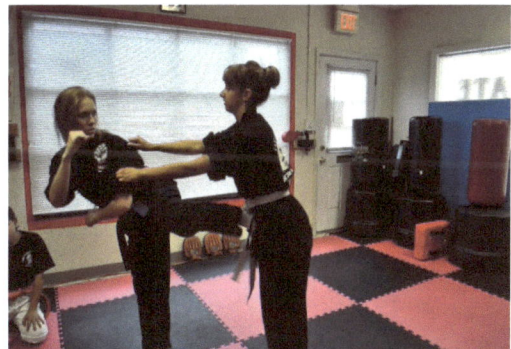

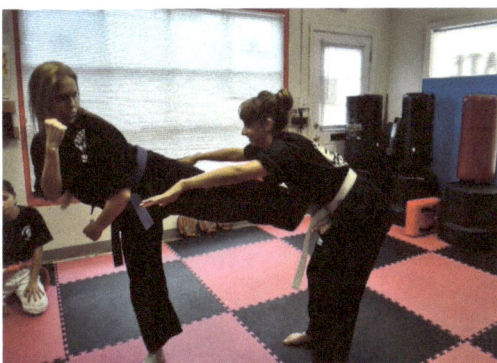

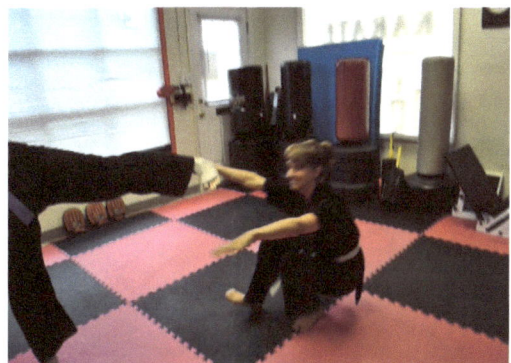

Here you will learn some Basic Striking and Kicking Techniques

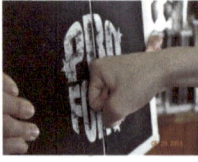 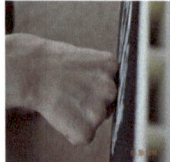

Punch using Two knuck-

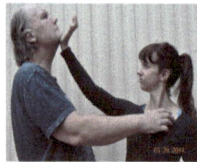

Palm Strike

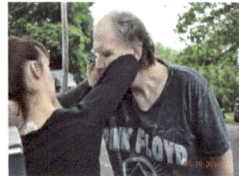 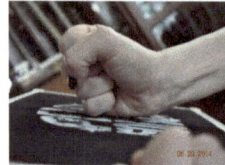 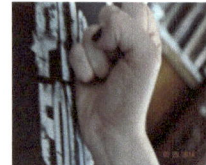

Elbow Strike   Elbow   Hammer   Hammer

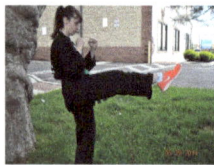 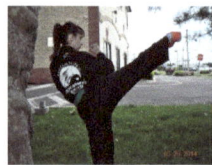 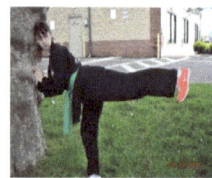

Front Kick   Side kick   **Back kick**

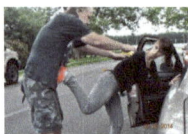 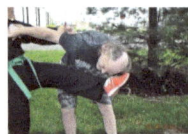 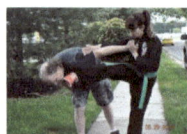 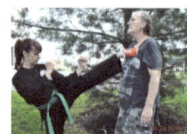 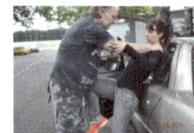

Back kick   Upward   Side Kick   Side Kick   Knee

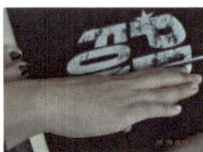 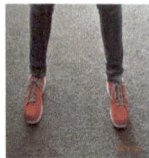 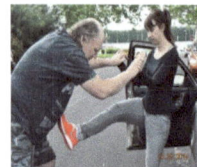 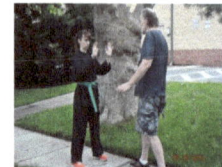

Ridge Hand   Stance   Front Kick   How to say STOP

<u>Aiki Jutsu</u> - Actual Self Protection Techniques
From a basic Grab.
<u>The Hand / Wrist Grab</u>

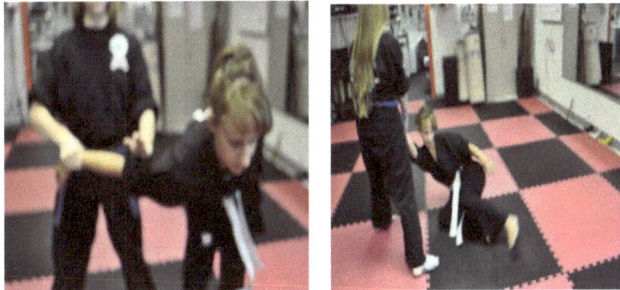

This is a Tactical Defense designed for an escape from an attacker. As with any grab, the thumb is what gives the hand all its strength!

Turn your arm against the thumb then grab their arm and turn over hold to keep in compliance.

<u>Cross arm Grab Escape</u> .

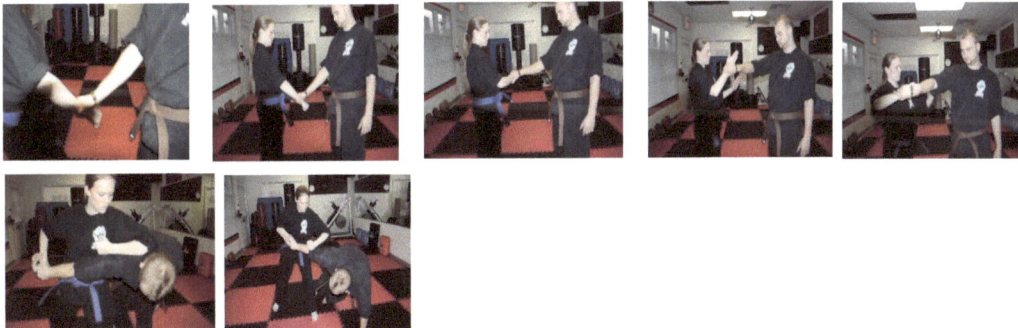

The adversary grabs your arm from across your body. The defender simply **lifts the arm toward the outside, gaining control of the situation. She then puts the adversary into a hold and strikes with an elbow strike to the base of the skull rendering the opponent unconscious, or you can just hold this position for a compliance technique .**

Here we have a choke Hold from the Frontal position

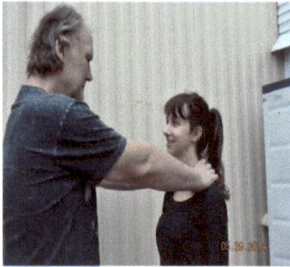

Pic. 1 the choke hold

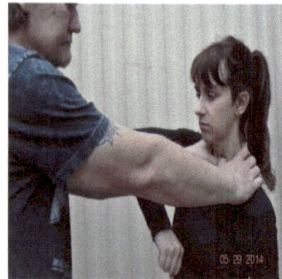

Pic. 2—take your right arm place it through the attackers arm grab your own hand

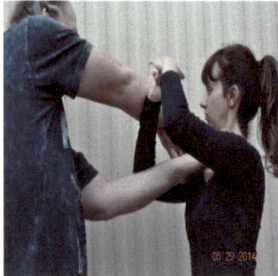

Pic. 3—next turn your arms upward with both hands until free

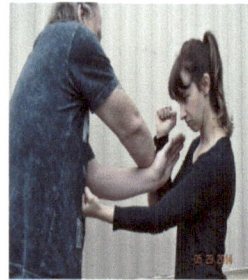

Pic 4– next you can now escape or add a reverse strike to the opponent s lower abs

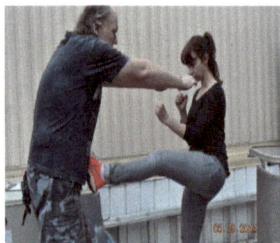

Pic. 5—you can now apply a Front kick if needed

Special Note : When being choked ,**don't panic** ,just hold your breath , you have plenty of time to escape this hold !Try to know your limit on holding your breath . Practice holding your breath for longer times. Once you know your max time , That's the time you have to apply any technique ! Don't rush it , be in control ! They will not expect your movement ,so don't give it away either!

Secret #7
The Choke hold from behind

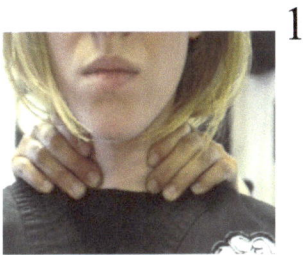

1

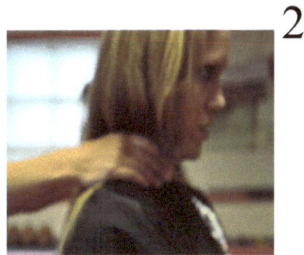

2

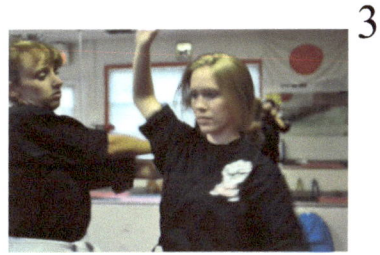

3

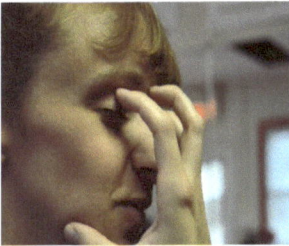

4

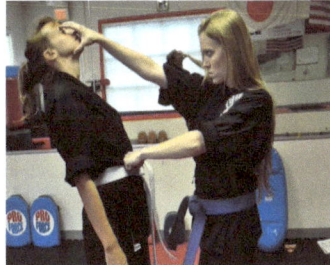

5

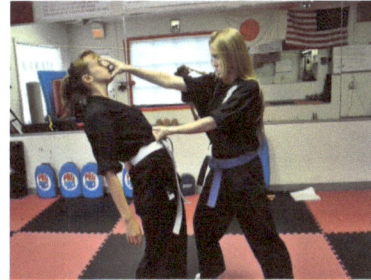

6

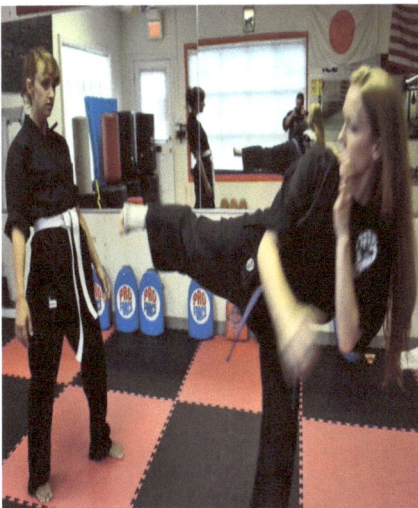

7

As you can see in pic. 1 and 2 the victim is in a rear choke hold position. She then lifts her arm and turns either direction. (pic.3) is ok, but make sure to know what is on your side! This lift and turn releases the hold and the victim is free! Then rake the eyes (#4) of the assailant as you strike. (# 5 &6) Then you may finish off with a kick in this final picture (#7). This a side kick.

This page is for more basic tech.
Like escape, push, shove !

Lapel grab or shoulder grab

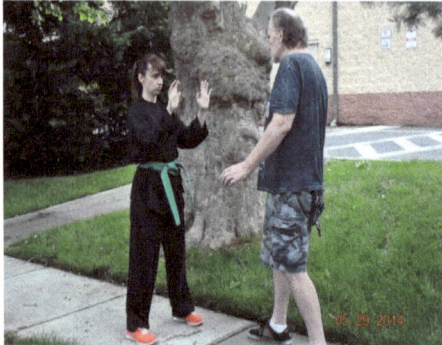

Here is the approach ,notice the stance and position of the Protection expert !

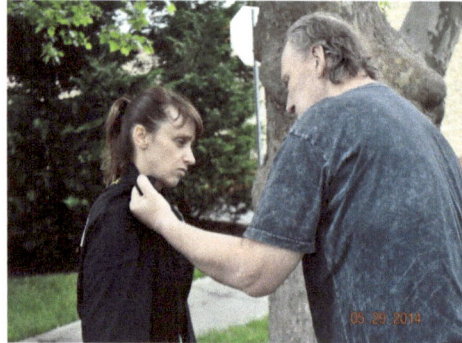

Here is the attackers grab as he vocalizes what he wants !

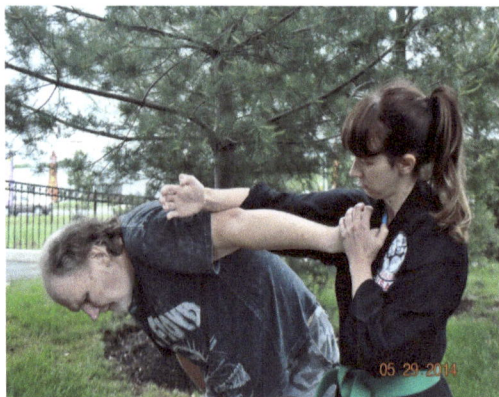

Turn the attackers arm over ,hold on with one hand then apply pressure on the nerve creating a pain full compliance arm bar !

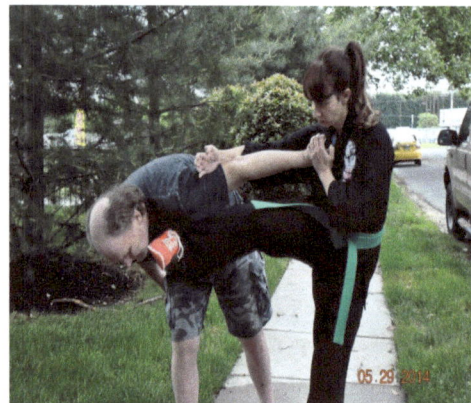

You may then add a side kick to the temple or lower jaw of the adversary !

Here are just a few pictures of myself with some of the most Legendary Martial Artist in the World.

KARATE

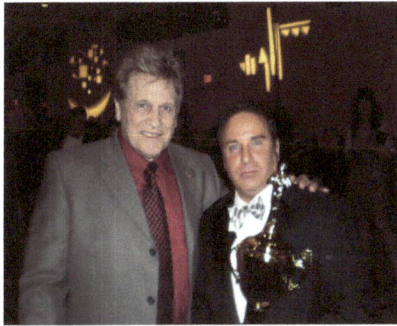

Joe Lewis
Undefeated World
Heavy weight Champion

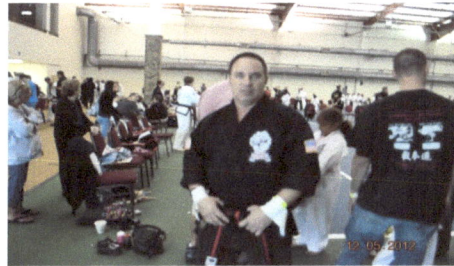

Charles Heimlich

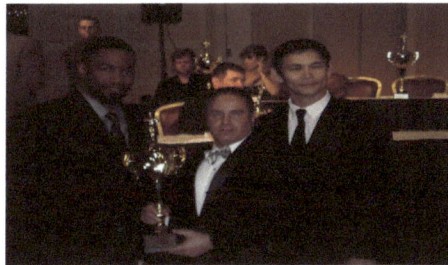

To my Left: **Michael Jai White**
Actor/ MA Champion /Celebrity
To my right :
Don "the Dragon " Wilson
World Champion/Actor/ Celebrity

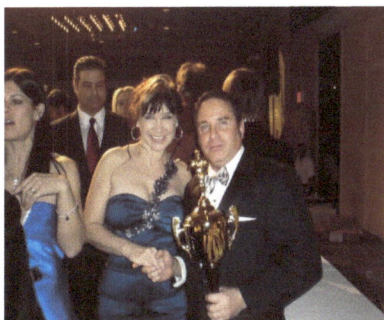

Cynthia Rothrock
World Champion /Actor /Celebrity

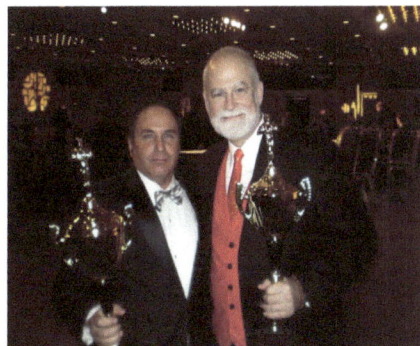

Steven Hayes

The Head lock

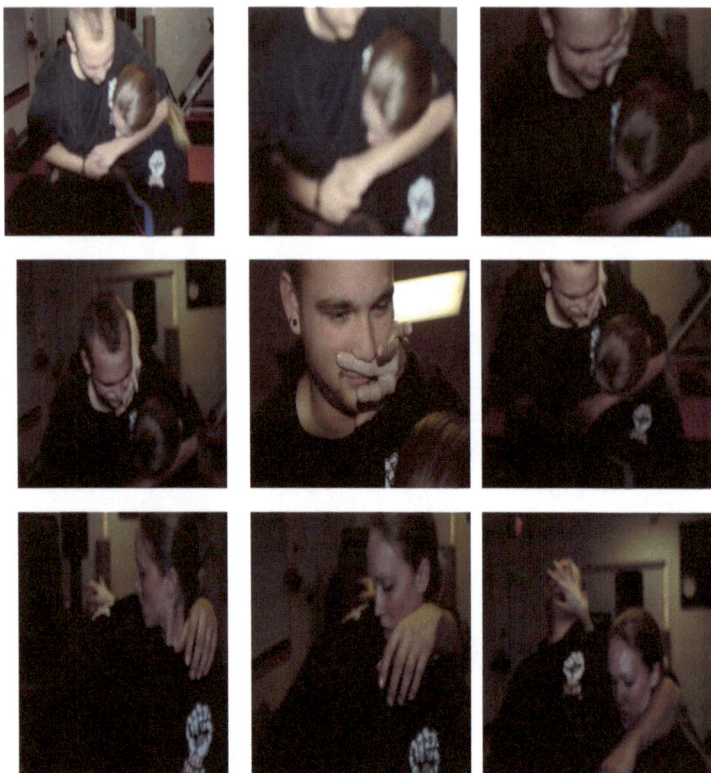

HEAD LOCK

In the picture on the left, the victim is placed in a head lock position. From the side in picture 4, the victim reaches around the assailant and places the middle finger on the philtrum located between the upper lip and the nostril. With a sweeping motion the assailant must let go and also looses balance. Now the victim may escape.

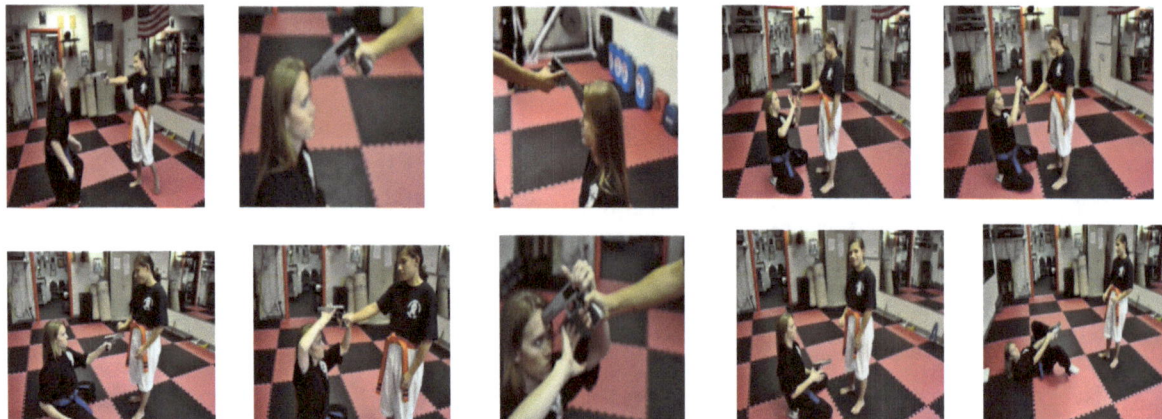

GUN THREAT EXECUTION STYLE

In this scenario, the victim is in a deadly situation. She faces a gun to her head in execution style. Though she remains calm, she reaches for the weapon. At the right time she leans slightly, rolls the gun toward the assailant. As she disarms her assailant she drops back to the floor with the weapon in her hand, then gives the command to the assailant not to move.

A Strike to lower jaw to stop your Opponent
Use good focus and control

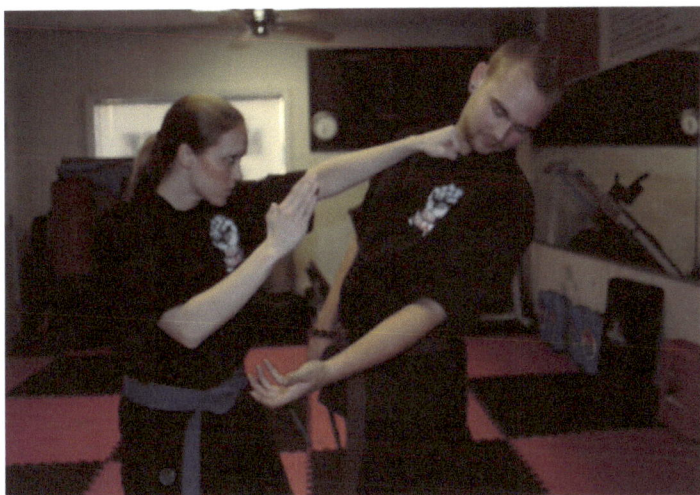

Grab control arm then add Elbow strike to back of Head

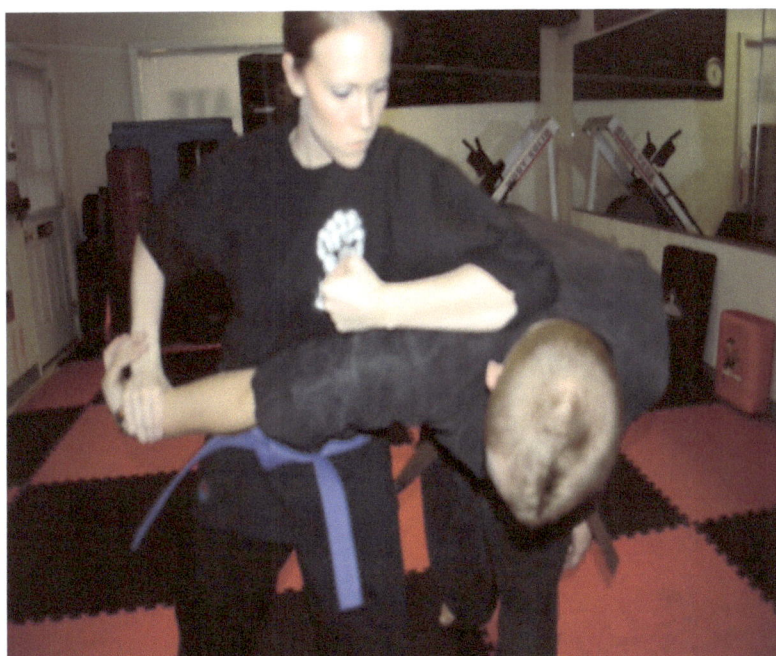

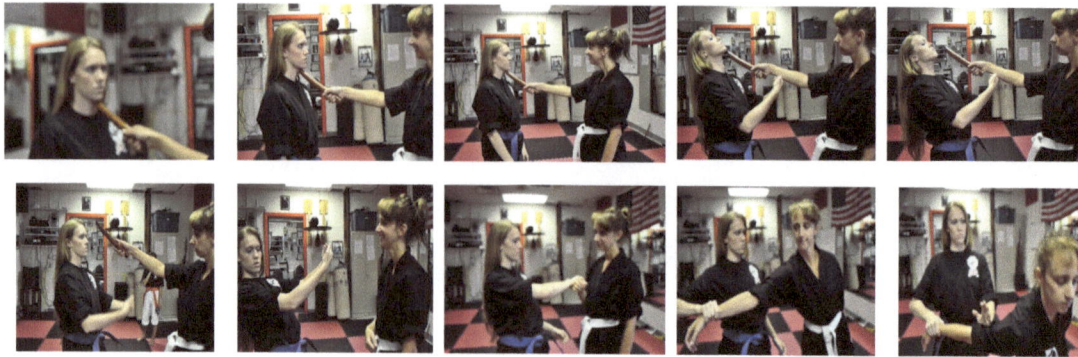

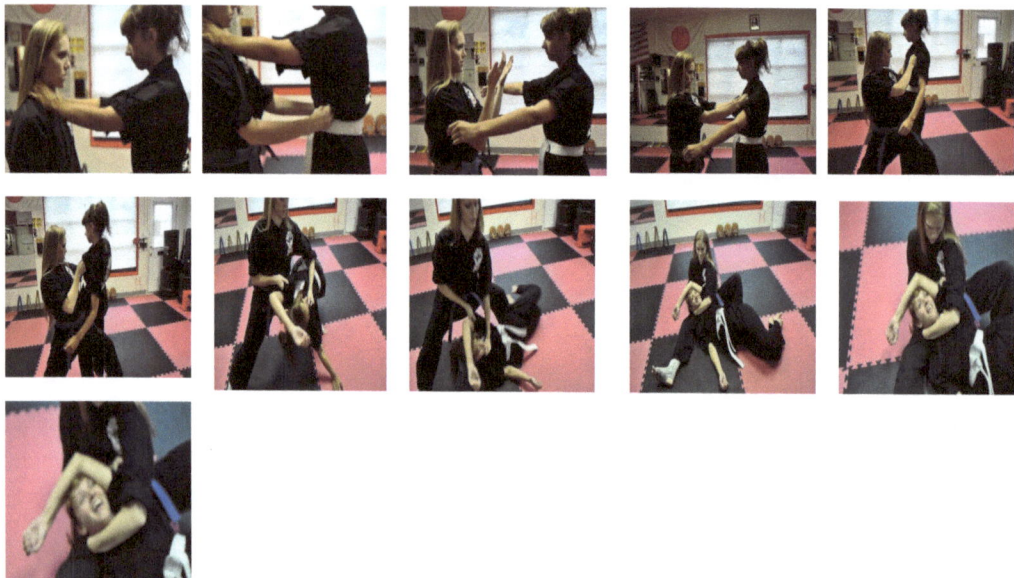

The top ten pictures depict a knife to the throat of the victim. As you can see the victim remains calm. She then creates a small space and therefore an opportunity to disarm the assailant.

In picture 4 she leans slightly and strikes upward hitting the radial nerve. Now disarmed , the victim gains control of the assailant's arm and stabilizes the assault.

In the next set of 11 pictures, we see an assault with a choke from the front of the Victim.

The Victim performs a double strike to the ribs. This loosens up the choke and gives the victim an opportunity to release the entire hold. She then grabs the assailant and steps behind to take down the assailant, and applies a finishing hold to the assailant.

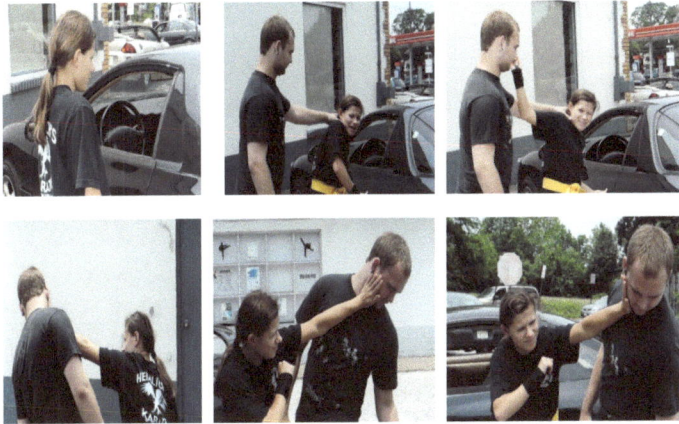

The victim is approached from behind. As she heads for her vehicle the assailant reaches out and grabs the victim. The victim quickly responds by turning toward the assailant while reaching out her arm to break the hold she completes the turn and throws a strike to the assailants jaw line .

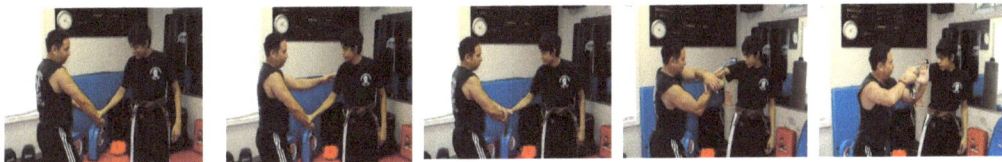

The HEIMLITRON being demonstrated here is a perfect choice for women as a personal protection tool . For one reason it is easy to carry , it is a key chain so it is discrete. Most importantly, it can not be used against you. Specialized training is required. Usually a certification seminar is mandatory!

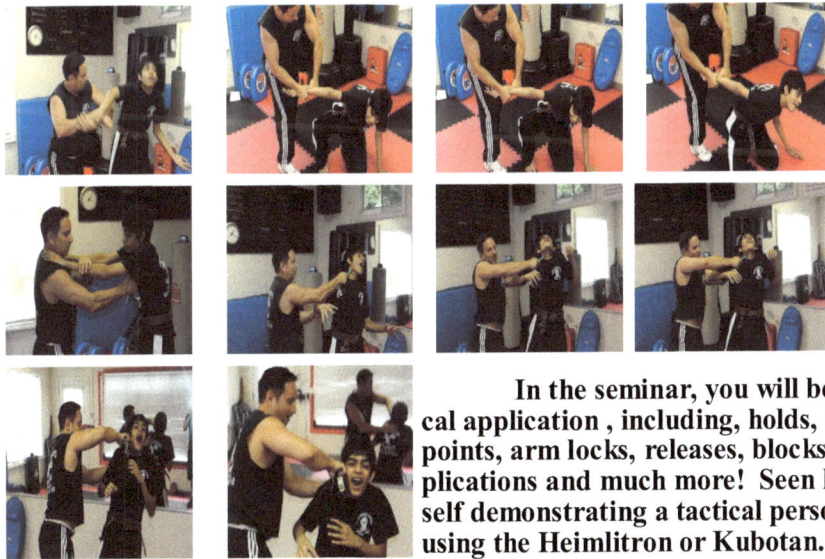

In the seminar, you will be taught all aspects for tactical application , including, holds, strikes, jabs, pressure points, arm locks, releases, blocks, controlled take down applications and much more! Seen here is Dr. Protection himself demonstrating a tactical personal protection technique using the Heimlitron or Kubotan. The pain you see on the opponent is real and left the opponent completely immobile with very little effort on the part of the demonstrator . Due to the more complicated applications in these pictures it is difficult to describe each series, therefore I will allow the reader to look at each picture and understand the application as they see it.

If interested in in certification please Contact Dr. Protection
Contact information is at the end of this book

On the next couple of Pages you will learn about basic Human Anatomy . Understanding Human Anatomy can and will give you better insight on Personal Protection ,for example, did you realize that at certain times of the day ,your body which is 78% water is effected by the tide?

During high tide you will bleed heavier and more forceful.
You need to be aware of this ,not only for your immediate Protection , but if you have to protect your self from a perpetrator while using a cutting type weapon, which again I do not recommend ,due to the fact they can take this away from you and use it on you ! Do not try this unless you have specialized training in order to be able to utilize a cutting type weapon with accuracy and precision , while having the understanding , commitment and responsibility that goes with this serious scenario. You must understand that you may have to take a life in order to save yours ! You must ask yourself , are you willing to accept and live with this fact ? It is mandatory for you to understand and know how to deal with this . You must teach yourself that you have this right that you deserve to live and thrive ! No one has the right to take this away from you and that you have the God given and legal right to take a life in order to save yours life or that of a loved one !

The human body has several vulnerabilities when it comes to self defense either with or with out a weapon, but when it comes to using a cutting type weapon here are some facts to remember .

1.-A cut to the **Brachial Artery** will result in a loss of consciousness in about 13 to 15 seconds and Death will occur in about one and a half minutes.

2.-A cut to the **Radial Artery** will result in a loss of consciousness in about 30 seconds and Death in Two minutes

Now lets examine some of the natural striking points that can be

Striking points of the Head

Top of the Head : At the very top of the **Cranial Vault** centered on the anterior two inches off the **Sagittal Suture .**

    The area where you would balance a book this is not always recommended it can put a serious strain on the neck however this is very effective when used in the right context .

Forehead : The striking point is the center of the **Frontal Bone**, about 2 inches above the eyebrow. This is the dome shaped structure in the front of the skull , and can receive tremendous impact without damage . Use this strike to the opponent's **nose , mouth , jaw or collar bone** , especially if the arms are pinned or bound .

Back of Head : The **Occipital Bone** in the area of the **Lambdoid Suture**

    This strike can be used when a assailant has you pinned from behind by ramming your head backward into the opponents **nose and mouth** can cause enough pain for a quick release .

Human Anatomy

There are 306 bones in the human body, of which smaller lighter bones only take about 10 to 12 lbs. of pressure to break.

There are 693 muscles in the human body. The strongest of which is the tongue and that's the one that causes the most trouble!

There are several hundred pressures points , of which ,we are only concerned with 365 for use in medical treatment or for personal protection. These points may be triggered in a certain order to obtain different results! Take note of this number!

Special Bonus!!! I will teach you an acupressure treatment

For medical healing.

Pressure Point #1
This is the headache point.
This can be found on the topside of the hand in the webbing between the thumb and forefinger. This must be triggered for 14 to 20 seconds. Bi Laterally Complete this two to three times, and results are immediate.

Pressure Point #2
Take your hand, place it at the wrist facing the thumb approximately four fingers away on the thumb side of the radial nerve. This is where the pressure point is located. Hold this pressure point for 30 seconds on both sides. This should be repeated 2 to 3 times until headache is relieved. Now this pressure point relieves migraine headaches, as well as regular headaches, in addition to pressure point number 1. It also helps with other difficulties.

Your Circle

PRIVATE SPACE = Distance x Space

This is the distance or circumference that goes around your body. A distance of approx. 3 ft.. A distance in which some one cannot reach you with a strike, kick, weapon, and they cannot grab you , even with a short step. This area is known as your safe zone and you must protect it as if it were sacred! For it is !

You have every right to stop some one from closing the gap, "as we call it" ,which means in simple terms, getting inside your circle. Once inside they are at a critical distance and you may be in harms way, so be careful not to allow this to happen! If someone does enter this space, you may tell that person to "STOP!", and, you may step back to keep the distance. If they have good intentions they will listen to your commands. They may even be some what apologetic. None the less a positive response you will receive.

If their intentions are not good, they will become irritated and argumentative and may resort to making you feel bad using guilt tactics. They will not listen and may even attack at this point. You must follow the Cue's, be assertive and find your boundaries. Do not give in and do not become argumentative! Do not swear or loose control! Simply ask them to listen to your commands and respect your rights as you prepare for the Fight or Flight Response in this situation.

The Mind, Eyes, and Voice

Your mind , eyes and voice are among your most powerful weapons.

Learning how to impede or intimidate your opponent with just your mind alone , may get you out of a threatening situation without any physical altercation. Learn to master this with the paralyzing look from your eyes ,and send terror to your opponent with sound of your voice !

When all combined they can devastate and temporarily disorient your opponent giving you the window of opportunity to escape or follow through with a strike or technique . Using your Voice , this special shout is better known in the Martial Arts world as the Kia , should not be underestimated!

When done correctly it can freeze an entire room of people! So practice this often and put all you have into it ! The Kia, pronounced (KEE- EYE) is a very effective tool It can also give you more sudden explosive strength ,which in turn gives you more power in your strikes or kicks making them that much more effective .You may want to incorporate this shout when practicing all your strikes and kicks.

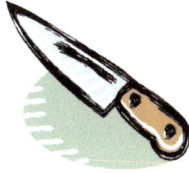

Can I Carry a Weapon ?

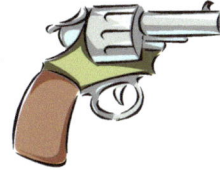

NO !

Self Defense weapons

First of all, I don't recommend women to utilize weapons of any kind! Especially a knife for personal protection with the exception of possibly two, The Kubotan / Heimlitron or Pepper spray. The Heimlitron is designed for women , but may also be used by Men . This is a keychain for personal protection and you must know how to use it! The other form of active personal protection is Pepper spray. This is very effective given that you again know how to use it. However, BEWARE , the pepper spray can be used against you where as the Heimlitron cannot. There are 5 types of sprays. They are ... The *Cone*, *Gel*, *Foam*, *Fog*, and *Stream*. The stream is the most recommended!

The Criminal

The Choice weapon by most criminals is the knife. The knife is deadly and can be easily concealed . It cannot be traced, is easy to get, and much more frightening or intimidating than a gun. However, Guns are becoming more and more common in recent years, and a lack of morals and values are the cause of the crime index rapidly increasing to such out of control numbers.

What do you recommend I use as a weapon ?

As I said before any thing can be a makeshift weapon, however , I recommend only two choices for you to actually carry with you and own beside a firearm ,(which carries a serious responsibility). If you do decide to invest and carry a Firearm, you must take certification courses, and learn proper use, care and the laws surrounding this type of Personal protection.

Here are the two legal choices that you can obtain relatively easily:
 First, is the Pepper spray which I discussed on the previous page!
 Next is the Kubotan, a basic Key chain self defense weapon! This is a weapon , that I believe to be one of the most valuable pieces of equipment in your arsenal , mostly due to the fact that most people do not know about this and don't know how to use it.

Now for a new and advanced weapon of choice, the Heimlitron, in development stages at this time will be the weapon of the future for many reasons, look for it soon ,it is similar to the kubotan, but much more advanced. When it hits the Market it will be a device to be reckoned with as well as a mandatory personal protection device .

I have added one Heimlitron technique so that you may see the immense benefits of owning this special unique personal Protection tool ,

see Kubotan or Heimlitron page!

How many main weapons does the Human body possess?

The answer is 9 basic they consist of the
feet, knees, hands, elbows and of course the
head. In order to use these weapons efficiently ,and effectively one must
train in the Martial Arts. Or have this book !

What is a make shift weapon?

For any Heimlich's Karate Student or my TNT trained students
in which you are one now . any thing and every thing you see or touch.
Such things as a lipstick cases, chairs, brooms, pens, books, or even paper,
Cell phones all can be used as a weapon. More on this in my next book

KIHON
Basic Material

Strikes, Kicks, Blocks and Stances, are the basic foundation of the
martial arts known as "Kihon", it gives the T.N.T. practitioner
additional tools for Personal Protection. As seen in the following pages

Stances

For personal protection we recommend a basic stance designed for balance but not to show any type of training, in other
words you never want to give away your position and the element
of surprise .You don't want your adversary to think you may not
agree or comply with them , this is your secret knowledge and the
widow of opportunity is on your side, this is what gives you the ex-
tra edge in a violent encounter , so take full advantage of this scenario , never try to bluff your way through any serious encounter !

Kihon continued :

How to do a personal protection stance

Stand with feet straight forward feet under the shoulders , knees slightly bent and weight equally distributed , this will give you balance and allow you to move quickly and effectively . Practice this stance often , with hands up, if facing a Knife or any Sharp instrument , turn hands palms toward your self , other wise you may have your palms facing the adversary .

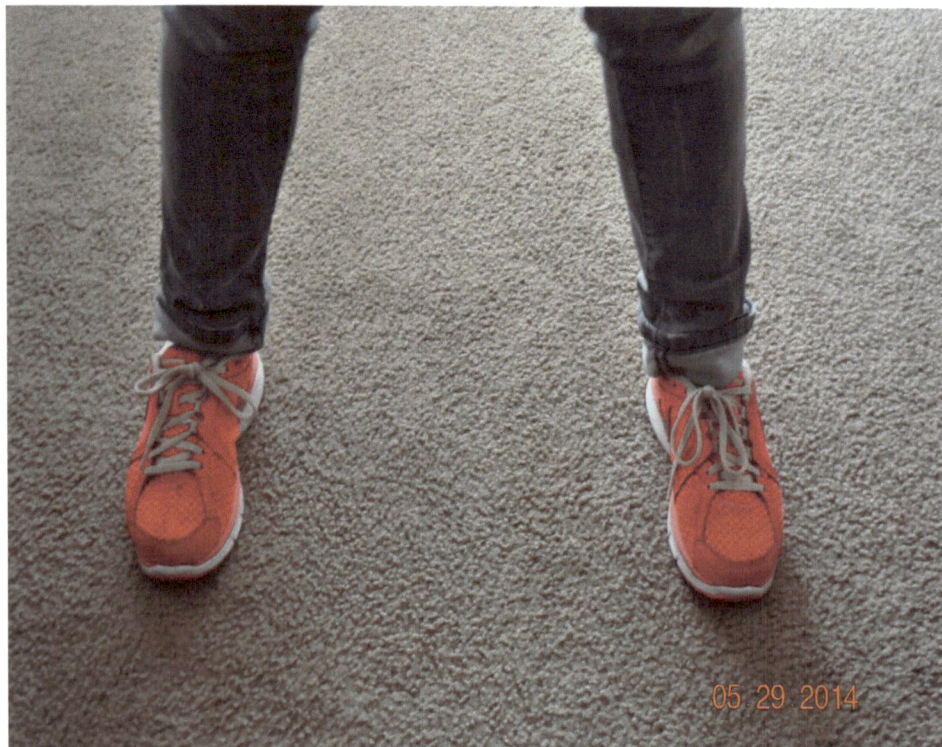

05 29 2014

Learn to step back with either foot at a slight outside angle from your Resting Stance when approached ,this will create more distance from your aggressor while setting up for your attack if needed . ALWAYS SHOUT STOP !   If in fact they have no true intentions on harming you , they will heed your warning . You must be stern and meaningful ! However if they do mean you harm they will not listen and may attack at that point ! Be ready to run when you can , if this is not possible then you will have to defend yourself ! This is where putting together all this material in this book becomes very critical you must train in all the lessons provided in this book and understand them know when to utilize a certain technique weather it be a strike a kick or even a block .

Then set up your next move , be it a grab or eye gauge ...be sure to always be aware of your surroundings and always look for a escape route . Never defend yourself against a assailant who has a weapon! You need to be able to get away to safety as quickly as possible . Never scream HELP .. You will most likely not get any . People will close their doors and blinds they for the most part do not want to get involved, but if you shout FIRE you will get the results you want ,people will come out of their homes they will approach you they will get involved and this maneuver will quickly change your situation .

In the following Pages you will continue to learn Kihon. Practice these strikes, blocks and kicks .As you learn them ,use proper form and execute them slowly with control ,build up your confidence ,then after you feel you have it together , you may begin to perform them at full speed and power ,but never losing control ! Practice on inanimate objects as well as on friends. This will build your confidence and set muscle memory in the movement once you learn all these techniques listed , practice them in combinations ,mix them up and put together routines ! This will enable you to follow up and follow through with multiple strikes and kicks for optimal Personal Protection . Remember quitters never Win and Winners never Quit! Be diligent Practice often , never stop training set up a time of day or a particular day ,preferably 3 x per week about 45 min is best, add this to your other workouts as well .

Kihon continued

How to perform a basic strike or (PUNCH)

Clench your fist very tight as you roll your fingertips down, clasp your hand with the thumb on the outside of the fist. Then only use the first top two knuckles on the thumb side to make contact, keeping the wrist straight, turn the hand slightly to the out side and tilted slightly downward , this is a proper fist , designed for contact. Begin striking soft targets and build up from there , I recommend a heavy bag for sticking and kicking as well as endurance training . Start with (6)-2 min. rounds build up to 12 rounds

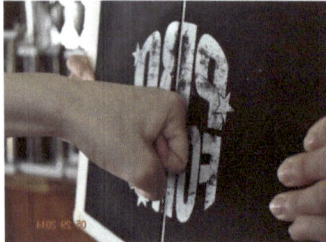

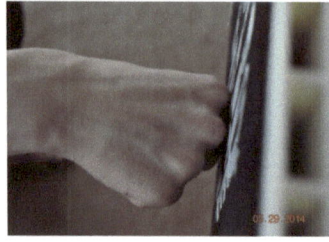

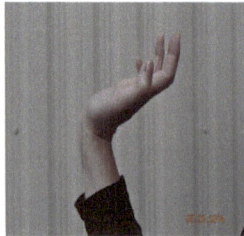

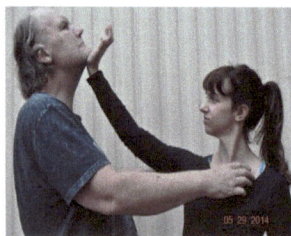

How to perform a open hand (palm Strike)

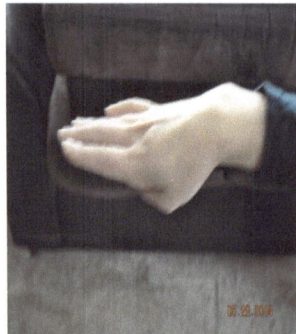

How to perform a ridge Hand or Knife hand

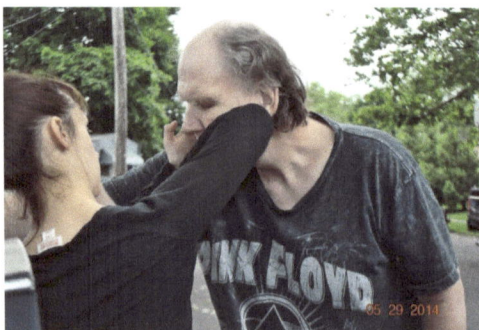

How to perform a basic inside elbow strike

Escape from a wrist grab

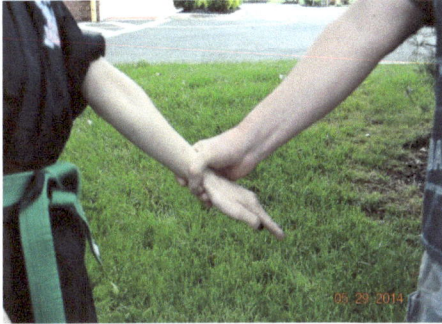

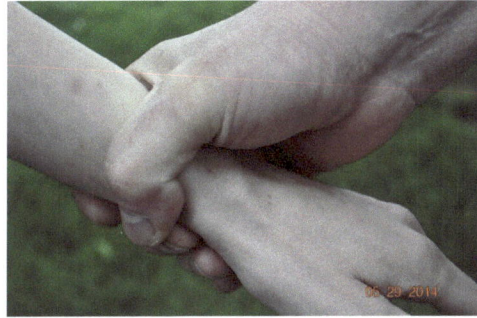

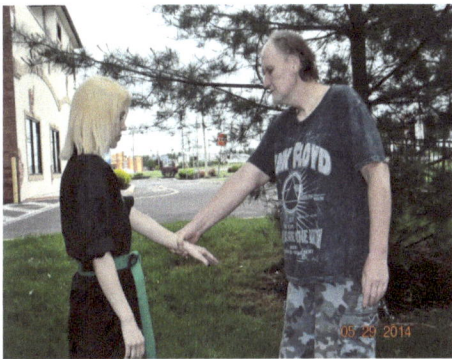

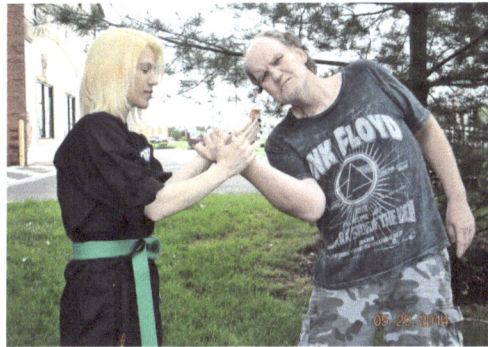

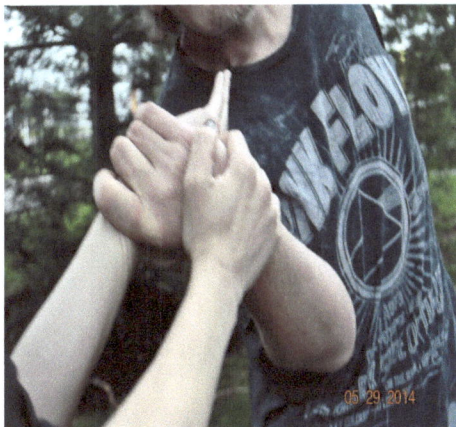

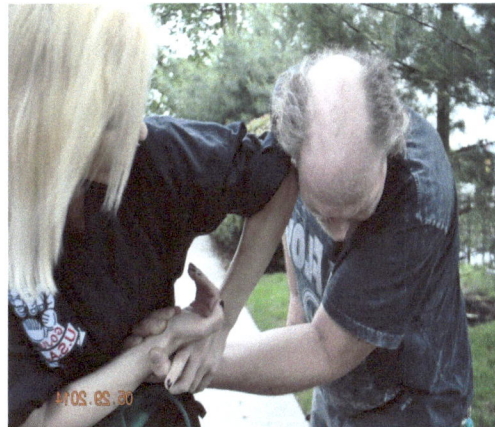

Turn the grabbed arm inward against the thumb until the grab is loose then using your other hand grab the opponent at the hand turn and elbow strike the opponent to the temple.

Kihon Continued

How to perform a basic front kick , pick up your leg keeping your leg folded tightly , then point your knee at the target , kick strait out keeping your foot flexed forward and pull the toes back exposing the ball of the foot , after contact , retract or refold your leg then place it down for balance, this will keep anyone from trying to grab your leg ,(I will not discuss complete stances or Blocks in this book).

Front Kick

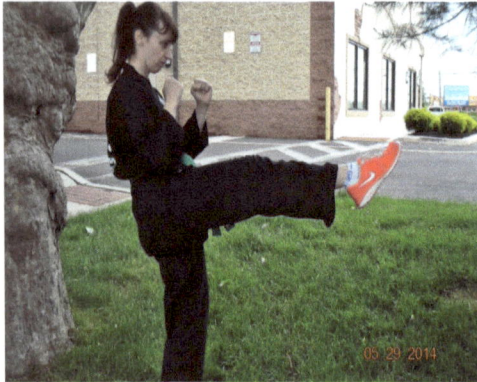

Front Kick applied

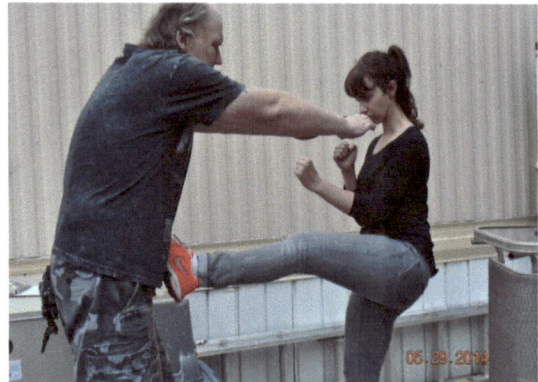

Side Kick

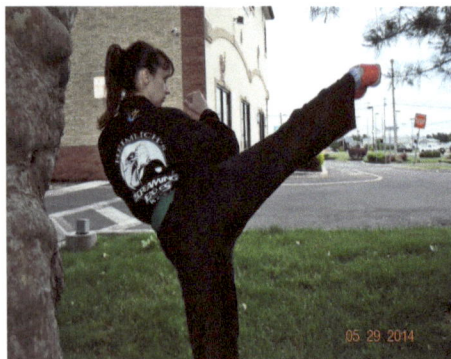

Side kick applied

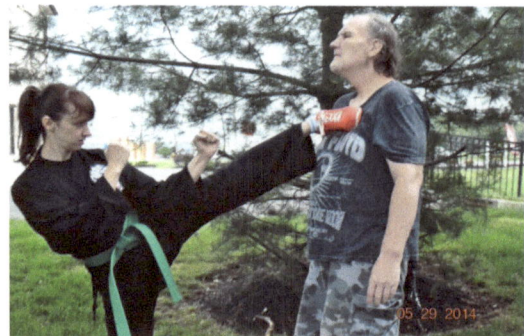

Back Kick

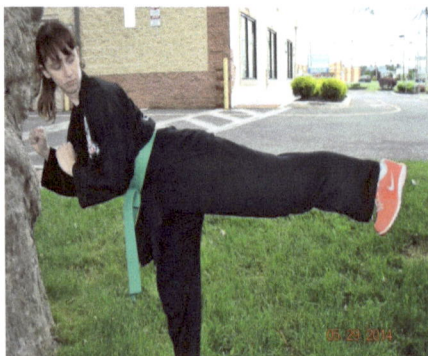

Back Kick applied

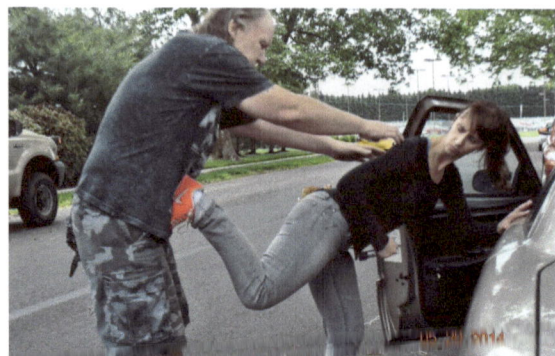

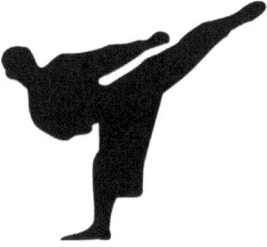

Protecting others .....

Well as if it isn't hard enough protecting yourself, protecting others is a whole different ball game. That is sometimes, or most times it is more complicated. Most people don't know what you know, and they believe they can assist you or help, when all they are is a liability.

People will sometimes try to intervene, which puts you in a more critical position.

So how do we deal with this?

First, If we are talking about your children, have an emergency protection plan. Use code words and special props. Have an emergency location or facility to meet at if separated. Remember to plan your work and work your plan! Set up mock scenarios and practice them often! Teach them self defense along with escape techniques and routes. Always travel with 3 or more individuals. If you must go out alone, act as though you are with a few other people. This will deter anyone that might have suspected you were alone. Keep your phone and keys out and handy.

If any one around you seems suspicious act as though you are on the phone with the police or husband. Also very important in protecting your family, is utilizing what I call a code word. A code word is a word or phrase that only a child and the parents know. This code word or phrase should be kept confidential and secret only to you and no one else. If an emergency ever arises, and you need to tell somebody the code word, then you will explain that code word one time. Then the child will know they can go with that person safely, because they know the code word. Otherwise they should never go. The child should never ask any stranger what is their code word. Also important in family protection, is staging. Make certain that your children know what is expected of them in case of an emergency.

Protecting others Continued

They need to know their role and need to know what to do. They should not hinder you in any way shape or form in providing safety. This can be accomplished a few different ways.

They could automatically know to go to the vehicle, lock the doors and stay there until safe. In the house there should be a safe room where they can go to and lock the doors. They should also know not to open it until a parent comes to get them They could go to a house near by, a family, a neighbor, a friend or a relative that they can go to quickly. If out and about and in a store, they can hide under clothes racks, and certain locations that have already been pointed out until the parent comes and gets them.

These are all safety related issues and very important for the parents to conduct. Make sure you practice with your child so they know exactly what they need to do. They cannot be argumentative in any way, you don't have time to argue. They have to do what they are taught to do immediately without question.

Your life and their life depend on it. If it is not your child we are protecting ,then be very cautious not to get involved , you may be getting in over your head and putting your life in jeopardy ! You may call for help or phone the Police , this would be the best way to help! Remember protecting others is not your responsibility, never feel obligated or guilty for any decision you must make!

You are Autonomous and you know your boundaries and limitations always be proud of who you are , never 2nd guess your self ! Just know that you did the right thing !

For more on protecting your children , check out our book Super Ryu Bee.
www.booksbyheimlich.com
Ww.heimlichskarate.com
Can also be purchased on Amazon

Use of force as it pertains to personal protection

Let me first say this ,

When it comes to protecting my self or my family and friends, I would rather be tried by 12 than carried by 6. With that said, it is very important not to abuse the right of personal protection! And make no excuses about it! You do have rights! However those rights must not break the law and the law states that the use of force must meet the act for justifiable use of force .

Use of force in defense of person:
A person is justified in using force, except deadly force, against another when and to the extent that the person reasonably believes that such conduct is necessary to defend himself or herself or another against the other's imminent use of unlawful force. However, a person is justified in the use of deadly force and does not have a duty to retreat if:

He or she reasonably believes that such force is necessary to prevent imminent death or great bodily harm to himself or herself or another or to prevent the imminent commission of a forcible felony

In certain situations, private individuals have the power to make an arrest without a warrant. These types of arrests, known as citizens arrests This occurs when ordinary people either detain criminals themselves or direct police officers to detain a criminal.

Citizens arrests are subject to fewer constitutional requirements than an arrest by law enforcement officers, but citizens arrests still have rules that govern them. Failure to abide by these rules can result in civil and criminal liability for the arresting individual.

Felonies

A person can arrest someone that they reasonably suspect of committing a felony, even if the felony didn't occur in the presence of the individual making the arrest. As long as a felony was actually committed and the individual making the arrest knew of the crime, a reasonable suspicion about the identity of the perpetrator will justify their arrest.

The felony must have actually occurred before an individual can make a citizens arrest. Even if a person reasonably believes that a felony has occurred, if the crime did not in fact happen, the person making the arrest could become civilly and criminally liable.

Breaches of the Peace

In general, people can't use citizens arrests for misdemeanors unless the misdemeanor involves a breach of the peace. Even in these circumstances, however, individuals can only make arrests when they have personally witnessed the criminal behavior and the breach has just occurred or there is a strong likelihood that the breach will continue.

Constitutionality of a Citizens Arrest

As mentioned above, a citizens arrest does not carry with it the same constitutional requirements that attach to an arrest by law enforcement officers. If, however, a person acts on the request of law enforcement, any arrest they carry out must meet the same constitutional standards as an arrest by the law enforcement officers themselves.

For example, a citizens arrest upon the request of law enforcement would still have to comply with the Fourth amendments restrictions against unreasonable searches and seizures and its warrant requirement. A citizen could also face prosecution under statutes that make it a crime to deprive someone of their constitutional rights.

If a citizen acts on their own initiative in making the arrest, however, those same constitutional restrictions do not apply.

Reasonable Force

Despite the fact that citizens arrests do not carry the same constitutional requirements as a typical arrest, individuals must only use the amount of force that is reasonable and necessary to make the arrest. Just what exactly constitutes the reasonable and necessary amount of force depends on the facts surrounding each arrest. Juries will usually examine the facts surrounding a citizens arrest and make the determination of whether it involved excessive force.

Some states prohibit the use of deadly force except in circumstances where the person making the arrest or someone else is faced with the threat of serious bodily injury or immediate use of deadly physical force. In these situations, the person making the arrest may use deadly force in order to prevent harm to themselves or others.

Other states allow people making a citizens arrest to use deadly force to stop a fleeing arrestee as long as the person making the arrest used reasonable methods in order to make the arrest. Some states go further and require that the person using deadly force first attempt to restrain the subject of the arrest, and other states require pursuit and an explicitly stated intent to arrest before using deadly force.

Any use of deadly force during a citizens arrest that does not comply with the applicable state law could result in manslaughter or murder charges against the arresting individual, as well as a **wrongful death** lawsuit from the family of the suspected criminal.

Tort Liability

In addition to wrongful death lawsuits, a citizens arrest has the potential to expose individuals to other kinds of tort liability if the arrest was not justified. If a person does not comply with the laws requirements when making the arrest, the arrestee could allege a number of offenses in a personal injury lawsuit, including the aforementioned wrongful death, <u>false imprisonment</u> and <u>assault</u> and <u>battery</u>.

Conclusion

Every individual is empowered to arrest wrongdoers in certain circumstances, but individuals looking to make a citizens arrest act at their own risk. Not only is the act of apprehending a criminal inherently dangerous, but failure to meet the legal requirements for a citizens arrest could have devastating consequences for the person making the arrest. Please look into your local Laws pertaining to this!

KNOW THE LAW!

Its your Right !

THE PSYCHE GAME

Do not allow yourself to be caught in a psyche game,
with anyone , much less a complete stranger! No matter how in-
nocent they may seem or look.
Remember, a coral snake is very pretty to look at but is deadly !

Never underestimate your assailant!
Remember they spend hours and hours every day honing their
technique.
They are always out and about and on the prowl.
Again I am not trying to scare you, but just to make you aware!

I don't want you to walk around watching over you shoulder
looking for a criminal.   I don't want you to panic at everyone
you see
But you must be more alert!   You must show strength and stabil-
ity at all times when out!

Never get into an argument!
Never look them in the eye unless contact is made
Do not allow someone the chance to start a conversation or to ask you a
question. You cant afford to be caught off guard. Now, there may be some
legitimate people out there that may indeed need directions , the time or
some other little tid -bit of information. You should however, remember
its your life, and its is not worth sacrificing for any reason. Its ok to seem
friendly, but not overly friendly and certainly not approachable. Do not
wear a watch out in public? Do not show off your jewelry? If you are single you may want to wear a mock wedding ring as a deterrent.
These little things when added up, greatly increase your chances and can
keep you from becoming the next obituary.

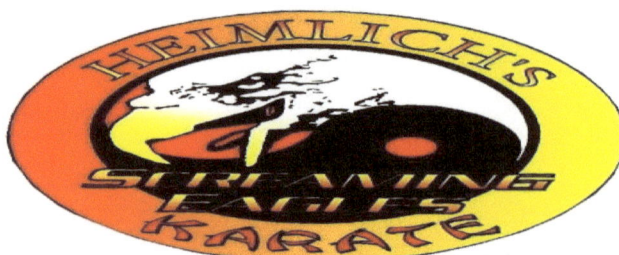

Listening to your instincts

We are all born with 5 basic senses

Sight , touch , feel , hear , and smell.
But we also have what is called a 6th sense,
Our Instinct!

We must learn to develop and listen to this primeval
Sense for it alone can save you life!

When you get an Eerie feeling about something, do not just ignore this
feeling, but listen and respond to it. Leave the unsafe area immediately!
This is a very important part of the arsenal of personal protection.
Sometimes you may get a queasy feeling in the pit of your Stomach. This
is the same thing. Its your instincts warning you of certain danger.

I can not emphasize enough the impact of ignoring this life saving sense.
I understand certain circumstances surround our efforts and puts us at
risk some of which are work, school events , groups, meetings, socials ,
friends, comfortable atmospheres e.c.t. .

Society today is caught up in a hurry up, get it done now attitude. However, do not allow this to ever interfere with your new dedication to your
Self ! You owe it to your self ! Its your right !

You have what I call the 3 rights.

1) The god given right 2) The legal right and
3) The personal right!

Understanding and excepting the reality of these rights
is your key to the Autonomy lock that sometimes
Bound us!

Common lures

One thing I must note in criminal awareness is, the fact that they use a very sophisticated array of psychological tools , which can detect your state of mind Body language, Walk , Talk, and a host of other indicators.

They are selective predators and will engage you in conversation in order to carefully evaluate fear, anxiety, and apprehension. They are looking for any weakness that tells them you are an easy victim .

So what do you need to be aware of ?

Some may simply walk up to you and begin what seems like harmless conversation, you show no fear and that you are not easily approachable. Another time they can seem to come from nowhere they may seem polite and helpful they will use guilt tactics to get what they want , be very cautious!

Some may act hurt and need your help, or ask you to put a letter in the mail box for them because they cant reach in from the vehicle . They may flatten your tire , then wait for you and approach you to see if they can fix it for you . Anther big one is unmarked police vehicles, if you are suddenly aware of flashing lights behind you and it is not an marked police vehicle do not pull over or stop keep driving you may call 112 this number can save your life .This number will call the State Police , you can ask if a real Officer is attempting to make a stop and can assist you from there. If you don't have a phone on you , then go to a very active place or a police station , this will deter them immediately !

So don't get caught off guard ! Always be alert! Know your surroundings !
Use common sense and good judgment ! If it doesn't seem right don't do it !

Another way they may distract you is to throw eggs at your windshield ! Do not turn on your windshield wipers, this will smear the eggs so that you can not see anything forcing you to stop. This is what they want to happen, then you are at their mercy I also advise my Students while driving never get out of your vehicle no matter what the commands are . When stopping at a traffic light ,give your self some distance from the car in front of you so that you will have an escape route if necessary .

These are just some examples of the lures that criminals use .They are very resourceful and can come up with ways to trick you and convince you . Don't fall for any of it ,remember they have all day every day to come up with methods to enhance their agendas . How many times did you feel someone was about to approach you, but then you thought you were wrong ? Well you weren't wrong , you were right but something you did changed their mind , that's what really happened . Learn from these things , study what's happening in the news, make yourself knowledgeable , and keep yourself safe !

Special Notes :

Kubotan or Heimlitron in use

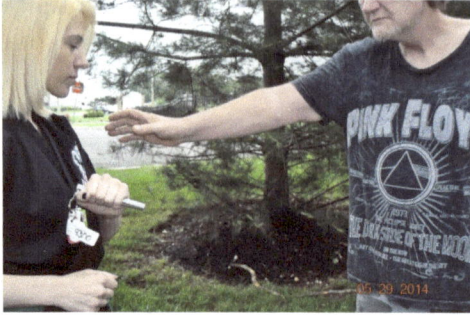

The opponent reaches for the victim

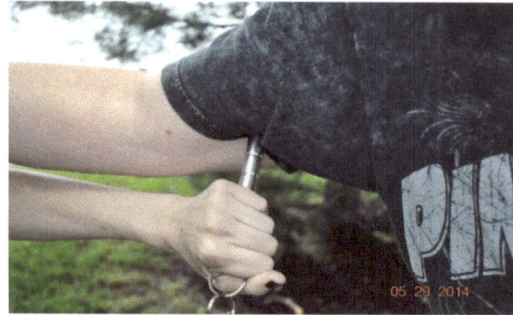

The victim steps toward the opponent and delivers a strike to the nerve just below the back of Bicep Muscle

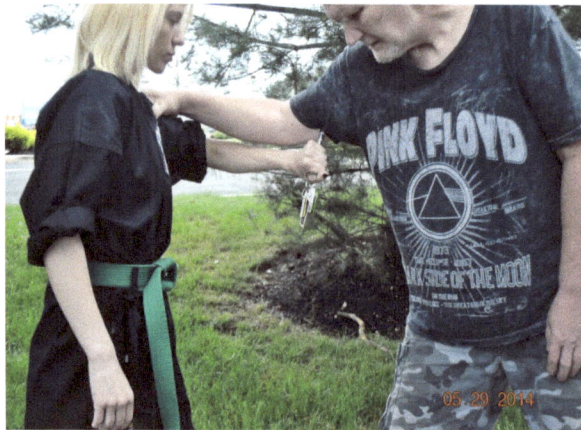

Same view

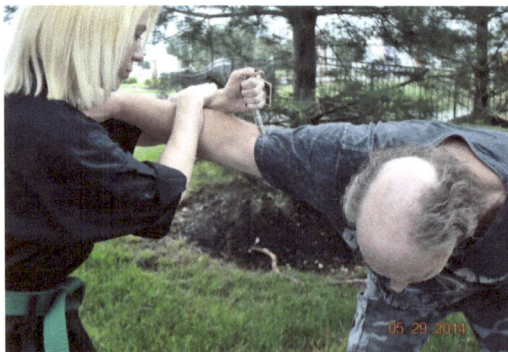

Reach over the arm from underneath and again apply pressure in the triceps tended causing the opponent to bend even more

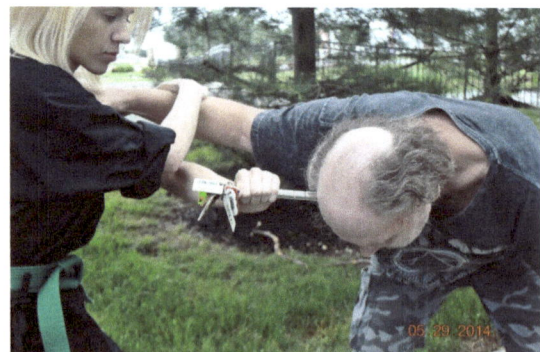

Now you can apply a strike to the Temporal lobes a final strike

58

Home Security

Many people are convinced that their home is safe, but what is safe? First of all, lets understand this, locks are made for the honest, and not the criminal. A criminal has great knowledge on locks. They understand how they can work and manipulate to open most locks quite simply, while others may give them a harder time. However, they will eventually gain access.

It is very important, not to rely on locks alone. Especially basic door knob locks. The dead bolt is the lock that provides the best security. However, make sure it is a high functioning, high security dead bolt double deadbolts for glass pane window doors are recommended. This will prevent the criminal from breaking the glass pane and simply turning the latch to gain access.

Window locks are not in itself a safe locking mechanism. They are quite easy to break, therefore I suggest a slide bolt action lock in addition to your basic window lock. In addition to securing windows and doors, I highly recommend some type of security system whether it be from an alarm company or basic home security surveillance cameras. Another important note is strategically home invasion techniques that include weapon placement, gathering area, panic room, as well as escape routes. A home invasion practice plan should be in place and practiced on a Quarterly basis. Children should be taught not to panic, they must do as their told, stay calm, not move, make no noise until either a parent or the police return to them. A part of the strategic escape route should include a neighbor's house to secure the family in a safe environment. This should always be taken very serious as home invasions have gone up dramatically in the past 10 years. Your home should be safe and secure. You should check windows and make sure you have double locks. Not just window locks but security locks as well. You can obtain those at any hardware store and having your own home security system is also recommended. Make sure a key is accessible, in case of a fire or an emergency, where you have to get out of your house, but keep both dead bolt locking mechanisms in the lock position.

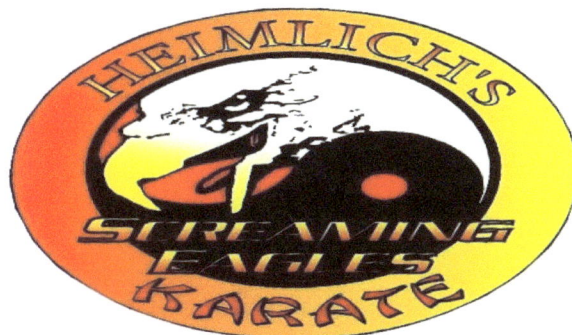

Home Security Continued;

Next, make sure you have a safe room for the children , your spouse and yourself. Make sure you have a strategic plan in your home if someone was to get inside your house. Can you lock them in the basement? Or other area keeping you and them separated so that you may seek Help !

Make sure you lock them away from you somehow? Do you have certain weapons set up inside? You can use a broom as a weapon, you can use a chair as a weapon, you can use any household item as a weapon. You can also use household chemicals , you can them spray in their eyes. If you do not have a gun in the house, make sure you have other make shift weapons available stationed throughout the house, and make sure you know where they are, and how to use them . Other security measures could be having a fold down ladder coming down from the second story window so that you can escape out of the house safely and securely. This is good in case of a fire or a home invasion. Make sure you have a place to go. This could be a neighbor's house or a vehicle. Have a key available at certain locations, that if you had to get out the house in an emergency you have a key for your vehicle. Keep your money strategically placed. Keep your valuables strategically placed. This completes home security.

I hope you learned many valuable lessons throughout this safety manual . Much of which will save your life ! Anyone interested in teaching my method of Personal Safety , can now do so , you will be certified according to our high standards , regulations and protocol , all of which must be Approved by Chief Master C. Heimlich himself !

Thank you ,

Follow my book to be better prepared and to ready for danger ,and to be able to be fully 98 % safer in the violent environment that we now all live in .Be safe my   friends .

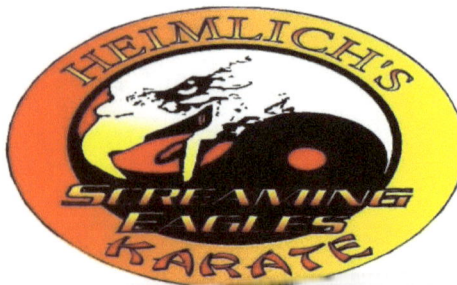

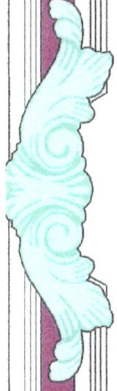

Master C. Heimlich's Personal Protection

Certificate of Completion

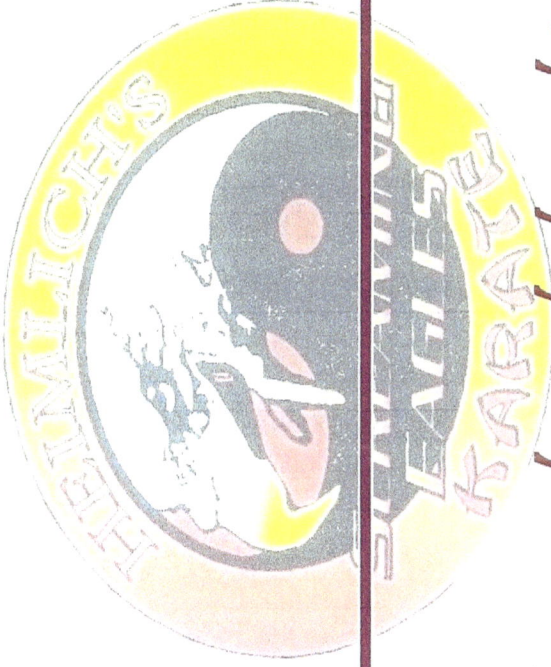

Has successfully completed the knowledge/understanding
of Personal Protection

Dated this   day of

Heimlich's Personal Protection for Women

Now different from many other books, this is not
THE END

This is actually just the Beginning !

Now take your new found education and put it to work!
The only time success comes before work is in the dictionary.
Remember the three rules of practice!
Practice , Practice and More Practice!

And by the way (NO!!!).... practice does not make perfect !
Only perfect practice makes perfect!
So now you may cut out your certification and complete the
information and Sign it you are now certified in Dr. Protection's
Personal Protection Safety Program . For information on how to
Teach our Program information on our Memberships
and other information or how to keep your certificate valid:
yes Valid it does have an expiration of one year and must be kept
up to date for authenticity you may choose from several options

Contact, : G.M. Charles Heimlich PhD
AKA. Dr. Protection
T.N.T. Personal Protection Safety Center
Heimlich's Karate
We are Dynamite
E– Mail drprotection@comcast.net
www.heimlichskarate.com
Also visit us on YouTube and Facebook
and all our other social media networks

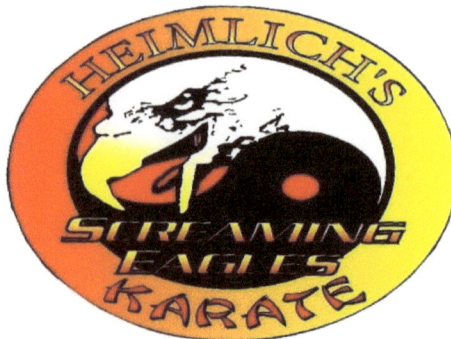